Preparatory
Manual of
Pathology

for Undergraduate Students

Preparatory
Manual of
Pathology

for Undergraduate Students

Sonam Kumar Pruthi MBBS, MD (Pathology)
Specialist
Department of Pathology
North Delhi Municipal Corporation Medical College
and Hindu Rao Hospital
New Delhi

———— Coauthors ————

Namrata Sarin MBBS, MD (Pathology)
Head, Department of Pathology
Hindu Rao Hospital, New Delhi

Sompal Singh MBBS, MD (Pathology), MBA (Hospital Admn), BSc (Statistics)
Senior Specialist, Department of Pathology
Hindu Rao Hospital, New Delhi

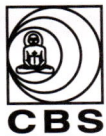

CBS Publishers & Distributors Pvt Ltd

New Delhi • Bengaluru • Chennai • Kochi • Kolkata • Mumbai
Bhubaneswar • Hyderabad • Jharkhand • Nagpur • Patna • Pune • Uttarakhand

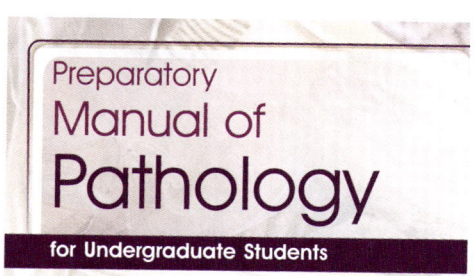

ISBN: 978-93-87742-80-2

Copyright © Author and Publisher

First Edition: 2018

Published by Satish Kumar Jain and produced by Varun Jain for

CBS Publishers & Distributors Pvt Ltd

4819/XI Prahlad Street, 24 Ansari Road, Daryaganj, New Delhi 110 002, India.
Ph: 23289259, 23266861, 23266867   Website: www.cbspd.com
Fax: 011-23243014   e-mail: delhi@cbspd.com; cbspubs@airtelmail.in.

Corporate Office: 204 FIE, Industrial Area, Patparganj, Delhi 110 092
Ph: 4934 4934   Fax: 4934 4935   e-mail: publishing@cbspd.com; publicity@cbspd.com

Branches

- **Bengaluru:** Seema House 2975, 17th Cross, K.R. Road,
  Banasankari 2nd Stage, Bengaluru 560 070, Karnataka
  Ph: +91-80-26771678/79   Fax: +91-80-26771680   e-mail: bangalore@cbspd.com
- **Chennai:** 7, Subbaraya Street, Shenoy Nagar, Chennai 600 030, Tamil Nadu
  Ph: +91-44-26680620, 26681266   Fax: +91-44-42032115   e-mail: chennai@cbspd.com
- **Kochi:** Ashana House, No. 39/1904, AM Thomas Road, Valanjambalam,
  Ernakulam 682 016, Kochi, Kerala
  Ph: +91-484-4059061-62-64-65   Fax: +91-484-4059065   e-mail: kochi@cbspd.com
- **Kolkata:** 6/B, Ground Floor, Rameswar Shaw Road, Kolkata-700 014, West Bengal
  Ph: +91-33-22891126, 22891127, 22891128   e-mail: kolkata@cbspd.com
- **Mumbai:** 83-C, Dr E Moses Road, Worli, Mumbai-400018, Maharashtra
  Ph: +91-22-24902340/41   Fax: +91-22-24902342   e-mail: mumbai@cbspd.com

Representatives

• Bhubaneswar	0-9911037372	• Hyderabad	0-9885175004	• Jharkhand	0-9811541605
• Nagpur	0-9021734563	• Patna	0-9334159340	• Pune	0-9623451994
• Uttarakhand	0-9716462459				

Printed at: Nutech Print Services, Faridabad, India

_to_

My loved ones

Foreword

Dr Sonam Pruthi, apparently of placid and quiet personality, but contrarily the most zealous and dedicated postgraduate student during his MD (Pathology) training and tutorship in Kasturba Medical College, Mangalore, Manipal Academy of Higher Education. It is my esteemed pleasure to write this Foreword to his second book *Preparatory Manual of Pathology for Undergraduate Students.*

In his endeavor to make pathology easier for MBBS students, Dr Pruthi undertook a humongous task to study several years' examination papers of various universities, and understood the commonalities, requirements and expectations of the examiners. His current book, which is essentially a preparatory manual for the undergraduate pathology examination, caters to all the possible questions asked in the theory examination. Hence, each chapter is presented in a question–answer format so that the student can essentially revise the entire syllabus in a short time span. The answers are elucidated in point-wise fashion as well as in an easily memorisable manner. His deeply entrenched passion for the subject is obvious in his efforts to maintain the language in the book as lucid but adhering to specific points or requisite matter an examiner would invariably look for while evaluating an answer paper. Whichever the format, that is long question, short answer question or short note, the student can attempt them comfortably and also score good marks. This worthy compilation is definitely going to fill the void of a good preparatory book in pathology and the students will be truly benefited.

His first book *Comprehensive Review of Pathology*, a collection of skilfully drafted MCQs, catering to NEET was received well by undergraduate and postgraduate examinees alike. Both the books if studied in tandem, will definitely enhance the understanding of the subject and make any examination a walk in the park.

My heartfelt best wishes to Dr Pruthi in this venture and God bless him with continuing success.

Dr Shrijeet Chakraborti
MD, DNB, PDF (Neuropath), PGDEA, MNAMS

Specialty Doctor (Histopathology), Leighton Hospital, Crewe,
Mid Cheshire Hospitals, NHS Foundation Trust, UK

Ex-Associate Professor and in-charge, Blood Bank,
Department of Pathology, Kasturba Medical College, Mangalore,
Manipal University, India

Preface

Book is written to make the subject revise fast during examination time, when there is very less time for revision and there is so much to read, and that too of all four subjects. During my MBBS days, I always used to think that if there could be any book which can save my time during university examination, because it becomes very difficult to revise standard textbooks immediately before examination and especially during the night of examination, in a short span of time, even if one has read standard textbooks many a times before.

Book is in question–answer format. Questions have been framed after going through the university examination of various medical institutions. Answers have been framed in accordance with the distribution of the marks of the questions being asked in university examination. Answers are written in a pointwise fashion, and points written are the one the examiner wants to read in the theory examination paper, so that one could gain more marks. Answers written cover the topic and wherever required flowcharts, diagrams, and histological figures have been added. Answers are explained in a simple language, which can be easily recalled at the time of writing your examination. All chapters of pathology are being covered in short possible number of pages, so that student can revise the content and fetch maximum marks. After reading the book, student will exactly know how answers should be written, which is tough when read only standard textbooks, so in that way, this book is going to make life easier during examination time.

Valuable suggestions, if any, to improve the book, are most welcome.

Sonam Kumar Pruthi

Acknowledgements

I would like to express my gratitude to my teachers, students and friends, especially Dr Rakesh Kumar Kalra and Dr Gulshan Rai Kuwatra, who were associated with me directly or indirectly, while writing this book.

I also want to thank my family for their unconditional love and immense support which cannot be exemplified with words.

Last but not the least, I also want to thank Mr YN Arjuna, Senior Vice President: Publishing, Editorial and Publicity, CBS Publishers & Distributors, and his editorial-production team for their hard work and effort, which made the publishing of this book possible in a short span of time.

Sonam Kumar Pruthi

Contents

1

The Cell in Health and Disease

Q1. Write a note on growth factors and its receptors.

Ans.

Role of growth factors: It stimulates the activity of genes that are required for cell growth and cell division.

Important growth factors and their role in cancers

1. *Epidermal growth factor (EGF) and transforming growth factor α (TGF-α)*
   ○ Two factors share a common receptor **(EGFR)**
   ○ **EGFR1 mutations** are seen in cancers of the lung, head and neck, and breast, glioblastomas
   ○ **ERBB2 receptor (HER2 or HER2/neu)** is overexpressed in breast cancer.

2. *Hepatocyte growth factor (HGF) or scatter factor (SF)*
   ○ **c-MET**—receptor for HGF is mutated in renal and thyroid papillary carcinoma.

3. *Platelet-derived growth factor (PDGF)*
   ○ Exert their effects by binding to two cell surface receptors, **PDGFR-α and PDGFR-β**
   ○ Stored in **platelet granules**
   ○ Stimulates hepatic stellate cells in **liver**, induces **fibrosis** and stimulates **wound contraction.**

4. *Vascular endothelial growth factor (VEGF)*
   ○ Includes **VEGF-A/VEGF, VEGF-B, VEGF-C, VEGF-D,** and **PIGF (placental growth factor)**
   ○ Signal through three tyrosine kinase receptors: VEGFR-1, VEGFR-2, and VEGFR-3
     – **VEGFR-1** plays a role in **inflammation**
     – **VEGFR-2** has **vasculogenic** and **angiogenic properties**
     – **VEGFR-3** induces the production of **lymphatic vessels (lymphangiogenesis).**

5. *Transforming growth factor β (TGF-β)*
   ○ It is a potent fibrogenic agent
   ○ Enhances the production of collagen, fibronectin, and proteoglycans
   ○ Inhibits collagen degradation by decreasing matrix proteases and increasing tissue inhibitors of metalloproteinases (TIMPs), thus leading to the development of fibrosis

○ **High TGF-β expression**—seen in hypertrophic scars, systemic sclerosis and Marfan syndrome.

Q2. Write a short note on fibronectin.

Ans.

Adhesive glycoproteins and adhesion receptors
○ Involved in cell-to-cell adhesion, and adherence of cells to the extracellular matrix (ECM).
○ Includes **fibronectin** (major component of the interstitial ECM), **laminin** (major constituent of basement membrane), **integrins** (cell adhesion molecules).

Fibronectin
○ Disulfide-linked heterodimer
○ Synthesized by fibroblasts, monocytes, and endothelium
○ Can bind to extracellular matrix components like collagen, fibrin, heparin, and proteoglycans
○ Helps in healing of wounds, in which it plays a role in ECM deposition, angiogenesis, and reepithelialization.

Q3. Discuss stem cells in detail.

Ans.

Stem cells: It gives rise to various differentiated tissues.

Two important properties of stem cells
○ *Self-renewal property*: Which permits the stem cells to maintain their numbers.
○ *Asymmetric division*: One daughter cell population enters a differentiation pathway and gives rise to mature cells, while the other population remains undifferentiated.

Types
1. *Embryonic stem cells*:
   ○ Present in the inner cell mass of blastocyst
   ○ Have limitless replicative potential and can give rise to any cell and hence are called totipotent
   ○ Can give rise to specialized cells of all the three germ cell layers.
2. *Tissue stem cells (adult stem cells)*:
   ○ Present in stem cell niches
   ○ Can produce cells, that are normal constituents of parent tissue
   ○ For example, hematopoietic stem cells, mesenchymal stem cells.

Examples of stem cell niches
a. *In skin*: Located in bulge area of the hair follicle, in sebaceous glands, and in the lower layer of the epidermis.
b. *Small intestine*: Located near the base of the crypt, above Paneth cells.
c. *Liver*: Liver stem cells (oval cells) are located in the canals of Hering (structures that connect bile ductules to parenchymal hepatocytes).
d. *Cornea*: Found at the limbus.

2

Cellular Responses to Stress and Toxic Insults

Q1. Define atrophy with examples.

Ans.

Atrophy
- Is defined as reduction in the size of an organ or tissue due to decrease in cell size and number

Examples
a. *Physiologic atrophy*: Seen in reduction in size of uterus after childbirth.
b. *Pathologic atrophy*: Seen in disuse atrophy (disuse of any organ), denervation atrophy (loss of nerve supply), diminished blood supply, inadequate nutrition, loss of endocrine stimulation, pressure.

Q2. Define metaplasia with examples.

Ans.

Metaplasia
- Reversible change in which one differentiated cell type (epithelial or mesenchymal) is replaced by another cell type.

Examples
- *Columnar to squamous*: Most common epithelial metaplasia.
- *Barrett esophagus*: Metaplasia from squamous to columnar type.
- *Connective tissue metaplasia*: Formation of cartilage, bone, or adipose tissue (mesenchymal tissues) in tissues that normally do not contain these elements.

Q3. Define necrosis. Discuss in detail with examples the different types of necrosis.

Ans.

A. Necrosis
- Occurs due to denaturation of intracellular proteins and enzymatic digestion of lethally injured cell.
- Due to damage of cellular plasma membranes, their protein contents leak out, which may elicit an inflammatory reaction.

Morphology

○ Necrotic cells show increased eosinophilia and have glassy homogeneous appearance.

○ *Myelin figures*: Large, whorled phospholipid masses, which represent damaged cell membranes.

Electron microscopy: Shows marked dilation of mitochondria with appearance of **large amorphous densities**.

Nuclear changes

a. *Karyolysis*: Basophilia of chromatin may fade.

b. *Pyknosis*: Nuclear shrinkage and increased basophilia.

c. *Karyorrhexis*: Pyknotic nucleus undergoes fragmentation and loss.

B. Patterns of Tissue Necrosis with Examples

a. *Coagulative necrosis*

○ *Cause*: Ischemia caused by obstruction in a vessel

○ *Site*: Can be seen in all organs except the brain

○ Architecture of dead tissues is preserved for a few days

○ Results in formation of eosinophilic, anucleate cells, which are removed by phagocytosis

○ *Infarct*: Localized area of coagulative necrosis.

b. *Liquefactive necrosis*

○ Characterized by digestion of the dead cells, which results in transformation of the tissue into a liquid viscous mass

○ Seen in bacterial or fungal infections and affects most commonly, central nervous system.

c. *Gangrenous necrosis*

○ *For example*, lower limb, that has lost its blood supply and has undergone necrosis

○ Represents coagulative pattern of necrosis

○ *Wet gangrene*: There occurs superimposed bacterial infection, resulting in liquefactive necrosis.

d. *Caseous necrosis*

○ *Caseous (cheese like) area*: Friable white appearance of necrosis

○ *Microscopy*: Lysed cells and amorphous granular debris with inflammatory cells, and a resultant *granuloma formation*.

e. *Fat necrosis*

○ Refers to focal area of fat destruction in pancreas and peritoneum

○ Occurs due to release of pancreatic lipases from pancreas in acute pancreatitis

○ Released lipases split triglyceride esters within fat cells, which combine with calcium to produce chalky-white areas (fat saponification).

f. *Fibrinoid necrosis*

○ Seen in immune reactions involving the blood vessels

○ Occurs due to deposition of antigen–antibody complexes and fibrin (that has leaked out of vessel wall) in the vessel wall

○ *On H and E stain*: The resultant deposit gives a bright pink and amorphous appearance, called "fibrinoid" (fibrin-like).

Q4. Discuss in detail about free radical injury, its mechanism and its pathological effects.

Ans.

What are free radicals?
○ Free radicals have single unpaired electron in their outer orbit
○ Reactive oxygen species (ROS)—implies oxygen-derived free radicals
○ *Oxidative stress*: Characterized by excess of free radicals

Free radical injury is divided in **3 phases**

1. *Generation of free radicals*

a. *Reduction–oxidation reaction* occurring during normal metabolic processes produces:

○ Superoxide anion ($O_2^{\cdot-}$, one electron), hydrogen peroxide (H_2O_2, two electrons), and hydroxyl ions ($\overset{\cdot}{O}H$, three electrons)

b. *Absorption of radiant energy*: For example, ultraviolet light and X-rays

○ Produces $\overset{\cdot}{O}H$ and hydrogen (H) free radicals

c. *Activated leucocytes in inflammation produce* $O_2^{\cdot}$

d. *Transition metals* such as iron and copper as seen in *Fenton reaction*

○ $H_2O_2 + Fe^{2+} \rightarrow Fe^{3+} + \overset{\cdot}{O}H + OH^-$

e. *Nitric oxide (NO)*: Converted to highly reactive peroxynitrite anion ($ONOO^-$), NO_2 and NO_3^-

2. *Removal of free radicals*

a. *Antioxidants*: Blocks free radical formation or inactivate free radicals, e.g. vitamin E and A, ascorbic acid and glutathione

b. *Enzymes* which act as free radical-scavenging systems:

○ *Catalase* (in peroxisomes)—decomposes H_2O_2 ($2H_2O_2 \rightarrow O_2 + 2H_2O$)

○ *Superoxidase dismutases (SODs)*—manganese SOD (in mitochondria) and copper zinc-SOD (in cytosol)—convert $O_2^{\cdot}$ to H_2O_2

○ *Glutathione peroxidase* (mitochondria and cytosol)—leads to free radical breakdown ($H_2O_2 + 2GSH \rightarrow GSSG$ [oxidized glutathione] $+ 2H_2O$) or ($2\overset{\cdot}{O}H + 2GSH \rightarrow GSSG + 2H_2O$).

3. *Pathological effects of free radical injury*

○ Lipid peroxidation in membranes, with resultant membrane damage

○ Oxidative modification of proteins, with resultant protein misfolding and breakdown

○ Lesions in DNA, with resultant DNA damage and mutations.

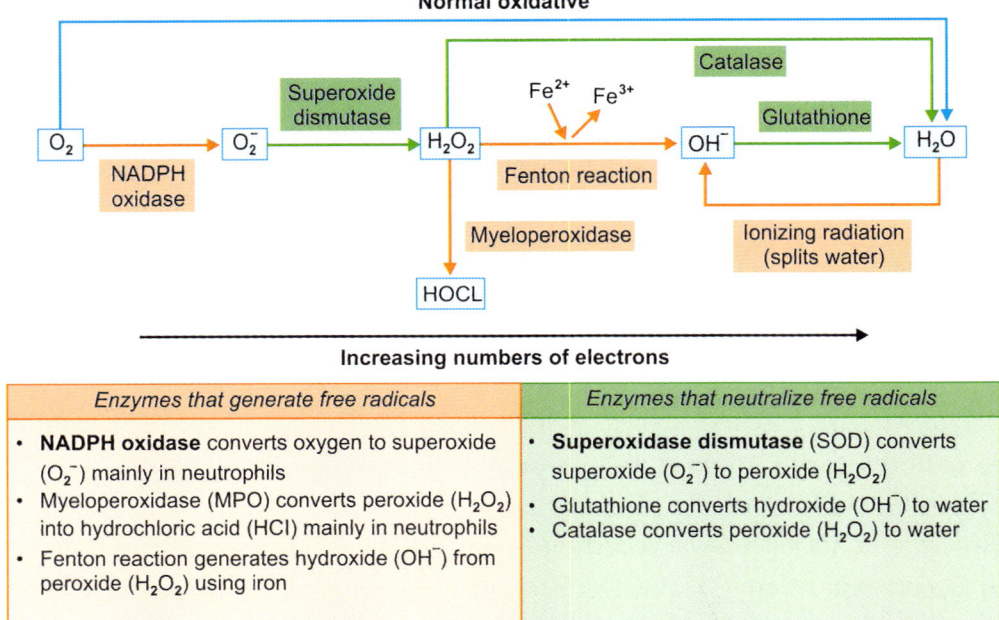

Fig. 2.1: Role of enzymes in generation and neutralization of free radicals

Q5. Define apoptosis. Discuss in detail the morphological changes, mechanisms, and examples of apoptosis.

Ans.

Definition: Programmed cell death in which the cells destined to die, activate intrinsic enzymes that degrade the cells own nuclear DNA and nuclear and cytoplasmic proteins.

Morphology
○ Cell shrinkage (cell swelling is an early feature in other forms of cell injury)
○ Chromatin condensation
○ Formation of cytoplasmic blebs and apoptotic bodies
○ Phagocytosis of apoptotic cells or cell bodies

Mechanism of apoptosis: Apoptosis results from the activation of enzymes called caspases.

Two Phases

1. Initiation phase

a. *Intrinsic (mitochondrial) pathway of apoptosis:*
  ○ Growth factors stimulate the release of anti-apoptotic proteins, which include *Bcl-2, Bcl-x,* and *Mcl-1*
  ○ In the absence of growth factors or when there is DNA damage, there occurs activation of BAX/BAK channel (as BCL-2 is antagonized), resulting in leakage of mitochondrial proteins cytochrome c
  ○ Cytochrome c (in the cytosol) binds to the protein called APAF-1 (apoptosis activating factor-1), which forms the apoptosome

○ This complex is able to bind caspase-9 (critical initiator caspase of the mitochondrial pathway)

b *Extrinsic (death receptor-initiated) pathway of apoptosis*:
  ○ Initiated by engagement of plasma membrane death receptors, which are present on variety of cells
  ○ Best known death receptors are type 1 TNF receptor (TNFR1) and a related protein called Fas (CD95)
  ○ The ligand for Fas is called Fas ligand (FasL)
  ○ *FasL* is expressed on T-cells that recognize self-antigens
  ○ When FasL binds to Fas, three or more molecules of Fas are brought together, resulting in formation of FADD (Fas-associated death domain)
  ○ FADD that is attached to the death receptors binds with inactive form of caspase-8 (caspase-10 in humans), via a death domain
  ○ Inactive form of caspase-8 and caspase-10 are brought into active form
  ○ Extrinsic pathway can be inhibited by a protein called *FLIP*.

2. **Execution phase**
  ○ Mitochondrial pathway leads to activation of the initiator caspase-9
  ○ Death receptor pathway leads to activation of initiator caspases-8 and -10
  ○ Both pathways lead to activation of executioner caspases, i.e. caspase-3 and -6
  ○ These enzymes cleaves DNA into nucleosome-sized pieces

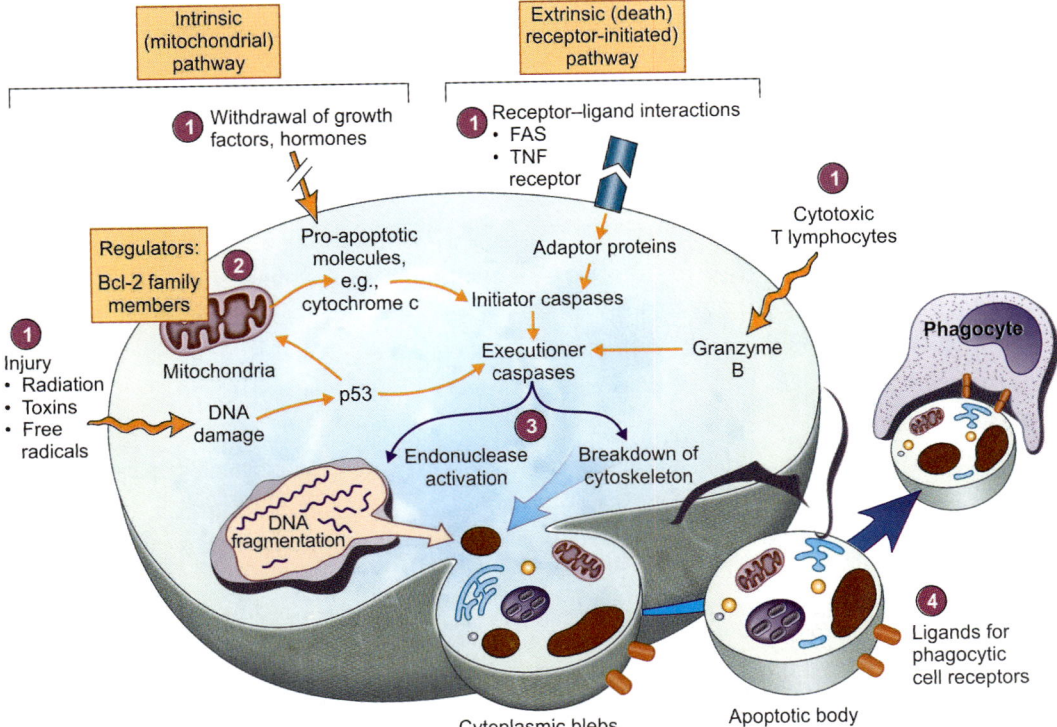

Fig. 2.2: Phases of apoptosis

Examples of apoptosis in health and disease

a. Growth factor deprivation results in cell death by apoptosis

b. *DNA Damage*: p53 stimulates pro-apoptotic proteins *BAX* and *BAK* with resultant apoptotic cell death

c. *Protein misfolding*:
- ○ *Chaperones/heat shock proteins (hsp70)* in the endoplasmic reticulum (ER) result in proper folding of newly synthesized proteins
- ○ *Unfolded protein response (UPR)*: Due to inherited mutations or stress, unfolded or misfolded proteins accumulate in the endoplasmic reticulum.

ER stress

- ○ Mechanism to handle unfolded protein response
- ○ Due to unfolded protein response, there occurs an increased production of chaperons
- ○ Chaperons reduce the load of misfolded proteins
- ○ If the above adaptation fails, cells activate caspases and induce apoptosis.

Q6. List the diseases caused by abnormal protein accumulation or misfolding of proteins.

Ans.

Examples of the diseases caused by misfolding of proteins: Cystic fibrosis, familial hypercholesterolemia, Tay-Sachs disease, Alpha-1-antitrypsin deficiency, Creutzfeldt-Jakob disease, Alzheimer disease, Huntington disease, Parkinson disease, Type-II diabetes.

Q7. Enumerate the differences between necrosis and apoptosis.

Ans.

Feature	Necrosis	Apoptosis
Cell size	Enlarged	Reduced
Nucleus	Pyknosis → Karyorrhexis → Karyolysis	Fragmentation
Plasma membrane	Disrupted	Intact
Cellular contents	Enzymatic digestion	Intact
Adjacent inflammation	Frequent	No
Physiological or pathological role	Pathological	Physiological (most commonly) or pathological

Q8. Write a note on necroptosis along with examples.

Ans.

Necroptosis

- ○ Characterized by *necrosis* and *apoptosis*
- ○ Morphological features resemble necrosis and mechanistically resembles apoptosis, hence called *programmed necrosis*

○ Triggered by TNF attaching to its receptor TNFR1

○ This mechanism is caspase-independent, but is dependent on signaling by the RIP1–RIP3 complex, resulting in cellular swelling and membrane damage as occurs in necrosis

Necroptosis is associated with cell death in:

○ Steatohepatitis (hepatocytic injury)

○ Acute pancreatitis

○ Reperfusion injury

○ Neurodegenerative diseases such as Parkinson disease

○ In host defense against certain viruses (e.g. cytomegalovirus).

Q9. Write a note on autophagy.

Ans.

Autophagy

○ Process in which a cell eats its own contents and triggers cell death

○ Occurs in a nutrition deprived cell, which survives by cannibalizing itself

○ The cellular organelles are now sequestrated into the cytoplasmic autophagic vacuoles (autophagosomes)

○ Autophagosomes fuses with lysosome to form an autophagolysosome

○ Cellular components are digested by lysosomal enzymes

○ Regulated by a defined set of "autophagy related genes" known as Atgs.

Q10. Classify pigments and write a note on Lipofuscin.

Ans.

Pigments

1. *Exogenous pigments*:
    a. Carbon (coal dust)
    b. Tattooing
2. *Endogenous pigments*:
    a. Lipofuscin
    b. Melanin
    c. Homogentisic acid
    d. Hemosiderin

Lipofuscin

○ Lipochrome or wear-and-tear pigment

○ Its presence indicates free radical injury

○ Appears as yellow-brown, finely granular cytoplasmic, peri-nuclear pigment

○ Seen in liver and heart of aging patients or in severe malnourished patients.

Q11. Write a short note on pathological calcification.

Ans.

Pathological calcification: Characterized by an abnormal tissue deposition of calcium salts.

Two types

a. *Dystrophic calcification*:
- ○ Deposition of calcium occurs locally in dying tissues
- ○ Serum calcium levels are normal
- ○ For example, seen in area of necrosis, in atheromas, aging or damaged heart valves and in tuberculous lymph node

b. *Metastatic calcification*:
- ○ Deposition of calcium salts in normal tissues
- ○ Seen in patients with hypercalcemia
- ○ Sites—interstitial tissues of the gastric mucosa, kidneys, lungs, systemic arteries and pulmonary veins

Causes of hypercalcemia

a. *Hyperparathyroidism*: Increased secretion of parathyroid hormone (PTH) with subsequent bone resorption

b. Resorption of bone tissue due to multiple myeloma or metastasis from breast cancer

c. *Vitamin D-related disorders*: Intoxication, sarcoidosis

d. *Renal failure*: Retention of phosphate, leading to secondary hyperparathyroidism.

3

Inflammation and Repair

Q1. Define inflammation. Describe the vascular and cellular changes in acute inflammation. Add a note on defective leukocyte function.

Ans.

Inflammation
- Host response that has the ability to get rid of the damaged or necrotic tissues and microbes
- Brought about by phagocytic leukocytes, antibodies, and complement proteins

A. Vascular Changes in Acute Inflammation

- Vasodilation: Mediated by histamine, results in increased blood flow, which causes erythema (heat and redness)
- Vasodilation is followed by increased permeability of microvasculature (occurs due to endothelial retraction or endothelial damage)
- Stasis: Dilatation of small vessels, packed with slowly moving red cells
- Neutrophils accumulate and adhere to the vascular endothelium, followed by movement into the interstitial tissue.

B. Cellular Changes in Acute Inflammation

a. *Leukocyte adhesion to endothelium*
- Normally, RBCs and leucocytes, flow axially, however, in inflammation, due to stasis, WBCs assume a peripheral position along the endothelial surface.
- This process of leukocyte re-distribution is called margination.
- Leucocytes adhere transiently to endothelium, detach and bind again, thus rolling on the vessel wall.
- Cells come to rest at some point where they adhere firmly.
- Rolling interactions are mediated by selectins {leukocytes (L-selectin), endothelium (E-selectin), and on platelets and endothelium (P-selectin)}
- Selectins and their ligands are regulated by tumor necrosis factor (TNF), IL-1 and chemokines
- Integrins: Bring firm adhesion of leucocytes on the endothelium

Integrins:
- Vascular cell adhesion molecule-1 (VCAM-1), the ligand for the β1 integrin VLA-4
- Intercellular adhesion molecule-1 (ICAM-1), the ligand for the β2 integrins LFA-1 and Mac-1

b. *Leukocyte migration through endothelium*
- Transmigration or diapedesis: Migration of the leukocytes through the endothelium
- CD31 or PECAM-1 (platelet endothelial cell adhesion molecule) is involved in the migration of leukocytes

c. *Chemotaxis of leukocytes*
- Leukocytes migration in the tissues toward the site of injury is called chemotaxis

Chemo attractants
- Exogenous: Bacterial products
- Endogenous: IL-8, C5a and leukotriene B4 (LTB4)

Defective leukocyte function
a. Leukocyte adhesion deficiency type 1:
- Due to defect in biosynthesis of the β2 chain shared by the LFA-1 and Mac-1 integrins

b. Leukocyte adhesion deficiency type 2:
- Due to absence of sialyl-Lewis X, the fucose containing ligand for E- and P-selectins

Q2. Write a note on phagocytosis.

Ans.

Three steps of phagocytosis

1. *Recognition and attachment of the particle to be ingested by the leukocyte*
   - Is done by phagocytic receptors on the leukocyte surface

2. *Engulfment*
   - Pseudopods (extensions of the cytoplasm) flow around the particle, resulting in the formation of phagosome, that encloses the particle
   - Phagosome fuses with lysosome, resulting in formation of phagolysosome and there occurs release of lysososmal enzymes

3. *Killing or degradation of ingested material is brought about by*
   - Lysosomal enzymes, reactive oxygen species (ROS, also called reactive oxygen intermediates), reactive nitrogen species, derived from nitric oxide (NO).

     Mechanism by which reactive oxygen species are generated:
   - Generation of ROS is due to NADPH oxidase (phagocyte oxidase), which oxidizes NADPH and, in the process, reduces oxygen to superoxide anion (O_2^-).
   - Respiratory burst: Rapid oxidative reaction, in neutrophils
   - $O_2^{\bullet-}$ is converted into hydrogen peroxide (H_2O_2)

- H_2O_2, in the presence of enzyme myeloperoxidase (MPO) combines with Cl^-, converting H_2O_2 to hypochlorite (OCl^-)
- HOCl is a potent antimicrobial agent that destroys microbes
- H_2O_2-MPO-halide system: Most efficient bactericidal system of neutrophils
- H_2O_2 is converted to hydroxyl radical (OH^-), another powerful destructive agent
- NO reacts with superoxide ($O_2^{\bullet}$) to generate highly reactive free radical peroxynitrite ($ONOO^-$), which brings microbe destruction.

Note:

- Reactive oxygen species are neutralized by **antioxidants** including superoxide dismutase, catalase, glutathione peroxidase, ceruloplasmin, transferrin

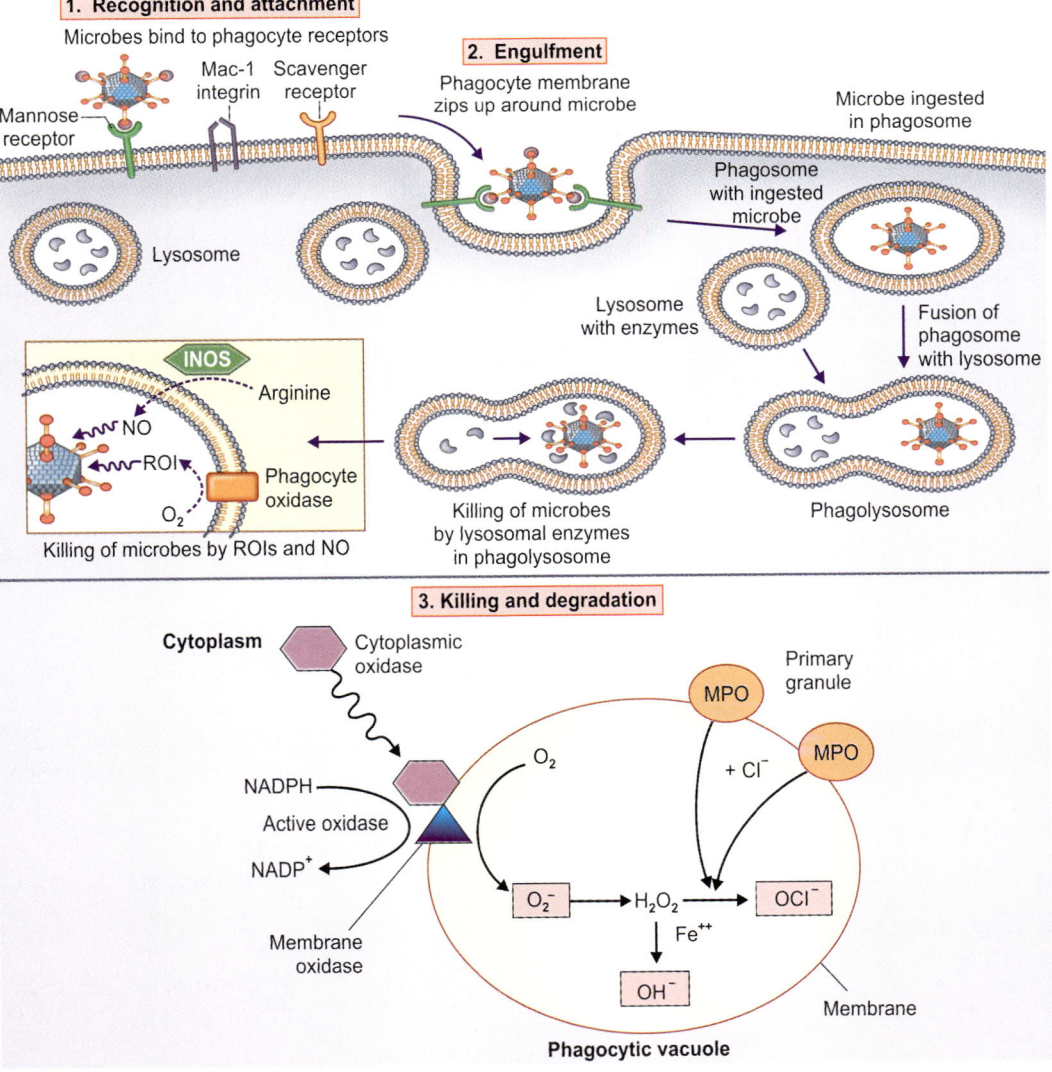

Fig. 3.1: Steps of phagocytosis

Q3. Write a note on chemical mediators in acute inflammation. Discuss the role of arachidonic acid metabolites in inflammation.

Ans.

Chemical mediators in acute inflammation:

1. Histamine

Release is stimulated by
○ Physical injury, such as trauma, cold, or heat
○ Binding of antibodies to mast cells (immediate hypersensitivity reactions)
○ Products of complement called anaphylatoxins (C3a and C5a)

Actions of histamine
○ Arteriolar dilation, increased permeability of venules, smooth muscle contraction

2. Serotonin (5-hydroxytryptamine)

○ Acts as a neurotransmitter in the gastrointestinal tract
○ Present in platelets

3. Arachidonic acid and its metabolites

Arachidonic acid (AA)
○ Normally present in membrane phospholipids, and is released by the action phospholipase A2
○ AA-derived mediators, are synthesized by cyclooxygenases (which generate prostaglandins) and lipoxygenases (which produce leukotrienes and lipoxins)

a. *Prostaglandins*
   ○ Produced by mast cells, macrophages, endothelial cells
   ○ Generated by the action of cyclooxygenase-1 and cyclooxygenase-2
   ○ Includes PGE2, PGD2, PGF2α, PGI2 (prostacyclin), and TxA2 (thromboxane A2)

b. *Leukotrienes*
   ○ Derived by the action of lipoxygenases enzymes

5-lipoxygenase
   ○ Predominantly seen in neutrophils
   ○ Converts arachidonic acid to 5-hydroxyeicosatetraenoic acid, the precursor form of leukotrienes
   ○ LTB4 is a potent chemotactic agent and activator of neutrophils
   ○ LTC4, LTD4, and LTE4 cause intense vasoconstriction, bronchospasm

c. *Lipoxins*
   ○ Generated from AA by 12-lipoxygenase pathway
   ○ Suppress inflammation by inhibiting the recruitment of leukocytes

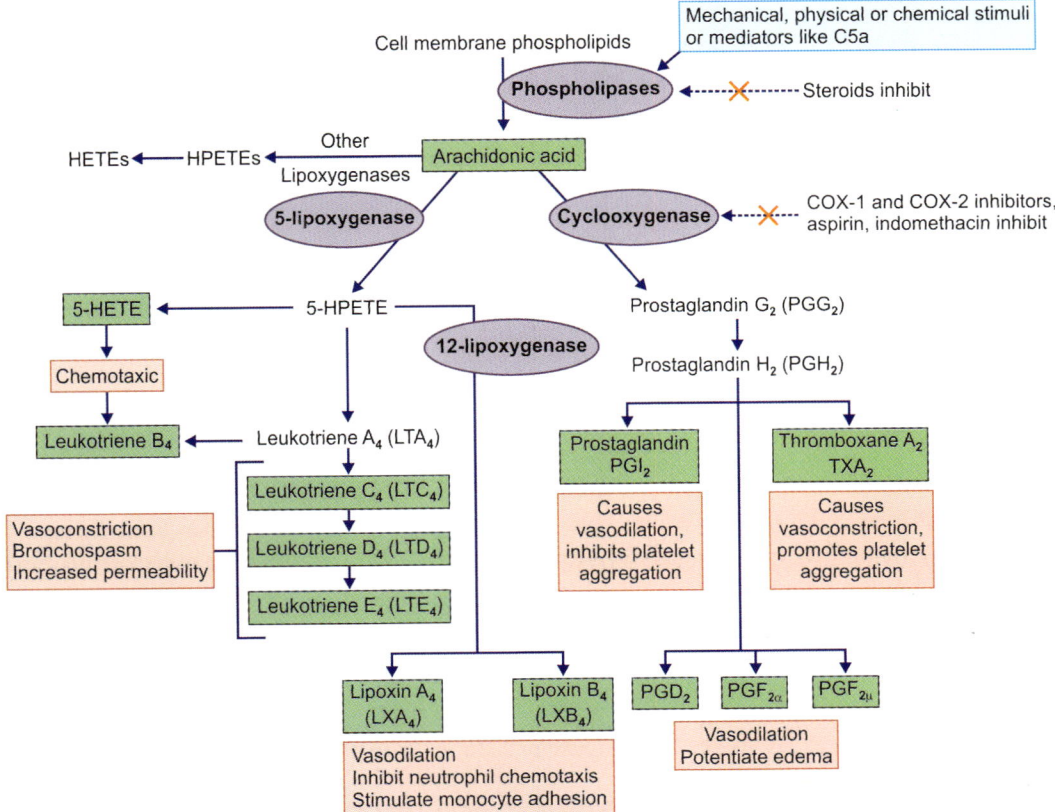

Fig. 3.2: Arachidonic acid and its metabolites

Q4. Write a short note on chemokines.

Ans.

Chemokines

- Acts as chemoattractants for leukocytes.

Classified into four major groups

a. *C-X-C chemokines* (α *chemokines*)

- Responsible for chemotaxis of neutrophils
- Secreted by activated macrophages, endothelial cells
- IL-8 is typical of this group

b. *C-C chemokines* (β *chemokines*)

- Attract monocytes, eosinophils, basophils, and lymphocytes
- Include monocyte chemoattractant protein (MCP-1), eotaxin, macrophage inflammatory protein-1α (MIP-1α), and RANTES
- Eotaxin selectively recruits eosinophils

c. *C chemokines (γ chemokines)*
  ○ Includes lymphotactin which is specific for lymphocytes

d. *CX3C chemokines*
  ○ For example, fractalkine
  ○ Promotes strong adhesion of monocyte and T-cells

Q5. Mention functions of complement pathway system.

Ans.

Functions of complement system

a. **Inflammation**
  ○ C3a, C5a are called anaphylotoxins, because they stimulate histamine release from mast cells
  ○ C5a-powerful chemotactic agent for neutrophils, monocytes, eosinophils, and basophils

b. **Phagocytosis:** C3b, acts as opsonins and promotes phagocytosis by neutrophils and macrophages

c. **Cell lysis:** Deposition of membrane attack complex (MAC) on the cells result in death of the cells

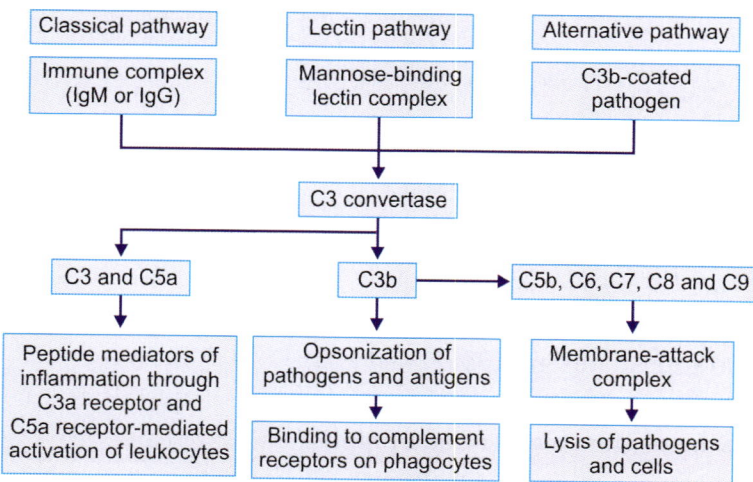

Fig. 3.3: Complement system

Q6. Write a short note on granulomatous inflammation.

Ans.

Granulomatous inflammation

○ Chronic inflammation, characterized by collection of activated macrophages, T lymphocytes, and central necrosis
○ Epithelioid cells: Activated macrophages with abundant cytoplasm
○ Multinucleate giant cells: Fusion of activated macrophages

Morphology
- Tuberculous granuloma has an area of central necrosis surrounded by multiple Langhans-type giant cells, epithelioid cells, and lymphocytes
- Central zone of necrosis (caseous necrosis) occurs due to hypoxia and free radical-mediated injury
- Can be seen in tuberculosis, sarcoidosis, cat-scratch disease, lymphogranuloma inguinale, leprosy, brucellosis, syphilis, mycotic infections, Berylliosis, reactions of irritant lipids.

Q7. Discuss systemic effects of inflammation. Add a note on acute phase proteins.

Ans.

Acute-phase response
- Systemic changes associated with acute inflammation.

Features of acute-phase response:

a. *Fever:* TNF, IL-1 stimulates the production of prostaglandin in hypothalamus.

b. *Elevated acute phase proteins:*
   - For example: C-reactive protein (CRP), fibrinogen, serum amyloid A (SAA) protein
   - Fibrinogen binds to red cells and causes them to form stacks (rouleaux), that sediment more rapidly and forms basis for measuring erythrocyte sedimentation rate
   - Prolonged production of SAA in chronic inflammation causes secondary amyloidosis
   - Elevated CRP levels is a marker of increased risk of myocardial infarction in patients with coronary artery disease
   - Elevated hepcidin (acute phase reactant) level is responsible for anemia associated with chronic inflammation

c. *Leukocytosis:*
   - Neutrophilia—seen in bacterial infections
   - Lymphocytosis—seen in viral infections (infectious mononucleosis)
   - Eosinophilia—seen in allergies and parasitic infestations
   - Leukopenia—seen in typhoid fever, viral, rickettsial, and protozoal infections

Note:
- Mediators of acute-phase reaction include TNF, IL-1, IL-6, type I interferon

Q8. Describe various stages of repair and healing and their abnormalities.

Ans.

Healing of skin wounds

a. **Healing by first intention or primary union:**
   Occurs in the following circumstances:

○ When the injury involves only the epithelial layer, epithelial regeneration is the principal mechanism of repair.

○ Healing of a clean, uninfected surgical incision approximated by surgical sutures

Changes brought about in the tissue include:

○ Within 24 hours: Neutrophils accumulate at margins

○ Between 24–72 hours: Granulation tissue is formed

○ Between 48–96 hours: Neutrophils are replaced by macrophages

○ End of first month: Scar formation

b. **Healing by second intention or by secondary union:**

○ Seen in large wounds, abscesses, ulceration, and infarction involving parenchymal organs

○ Repair process involves a combination of regeneration and scarring

○ Much larger granulation tissue is formed

○ Wound contraction is brought about by myofibroblasts

Abnormalities in tissue repair include:

○ Wound dehiscence and ulceration: Inadequate formation of granulation tissue or a scar

○ Hypertrophic scars and keloids: Excessive formation of components of the repair

○ Contractures: Seen on palms, soles, and anterior aspect of thorax, after serious burns

○ Exuberant granulation tissue (proud flesh)

Q9. Discuss the factors influencing wound healing.

Ans.

Factors that influence tissue repair

a. *Local factors:*

○ Infection: Most important cause of delay in healing

○ Mechanical factors: Early motion of wounds and increased local pressure, delay wound healing

○ Foreign bodies: Sutures, steel, glass, bone can impede healing

○ Size, location and type of wound: Highly vascularized tissues heal faster

b. *Systemic factors:*

○ Diabetes: Results in impaired wound healing

○ Nutritional status: Vitamin C deficiency inhibits collagen synthesis

○ Glucocorticoids (steroids): Weakens the scar due to inhibition of TGF-β

○ Poor perfusion: Due to arteriosclerosis and diabetes, impairs wound healing

Q10. Discuss the role of vitamin C in wound healing.

Ans.

Vitamin C

○ Results in activation of prolyl hydroxylases and lysyl hydroxylases from their inactive precursors, and the resultant hydroxylation of procollagen

○ Deficiency results in weak collagen chains

○ Weak collagen chains are inadequately cross-linked, lack tensile strength, and are more soluble and vulnerable to enzymatic degradation

○ As a result, there occurs impaired collagen formation, which brings about:

    a. Increased bleeding tendency

    b. Inadequate synthesis of osteoid

    c. Impaired wound healing

4

Hemodynamic Disorders

Q1. Define and classify edema. Discuss etiopathogenesis and pathology of various types of edema with examples.

Ans.

Edema is defined as abnormal increase in interstitial fluid within tissues.

Edema fluid can be transudate or exudate

○ **Transudate**—protein-poor fluid due to **increased hydrostatic pressure** or **reduced plasma proteins**, e.g. **heart failure, renal failure, hepatic failure**, **malnutrition**

○ Transudative effusions are usually translucent and straw-colored

○ **Exudate**—**inflammatory edema** (protein-rich fluid that occurs as a result of **increased vascular permeability**)

○ Exudative effusions are often cloudy due to the presence of white cells

Etio-pathogenesis of edema

1. Increased hydrostatic pressure
2. Reduced plasma osmotic pressure
3. Lymphatic obstruction
4. Sodium retention
5. Inflammation

Pathology of various types of edema

1. *Increased hydrostatic pressure* can be due to:
   a. *Impaired venous return*: Congestive heart failure, constrictive pericarditis, ascitis (liver cirrhosis), venous obstruction or compression, thrombosis, external pressure (e.g. mass), lower extremity inactivity with prolonged dependency
   b. *Arteriolar dilation: Heat, neurohumoral dysregulation*
2. **Reduced plasma osmotic pressure** (hypoproteinemia) can be due to:
   ○ Protein-losing glomerulopathies (nephrotic syndrome), liver cirrhosis (ascitis), malnutrition, protein-losing gastroenteropathy
3. **Lymphatic obstruction** can be due to
   ○ Inflammatory, neoplastic, post-surgical, post-irradiation

4. **Sodium retention** occurs due to
   ○ Excessive salt intake with renal insufficiency, increased tubular reabsorption of sodium, renal hypoperfusion, increased renin-angiotensin-aldosterone secretion
5. **Inflammation:** Acute inflammation, chronic inflammation, angiogenesis.

Q2. Discuss in brief, the normal mechanisms involved in hemostasis.

Ans.

Sequence of events leading to hemostasis at a site of vascular injury

a. **Arteriolar vasoconstriction:**
   ○ Brought about by endothelial cell injury
   ○ Due to stimulation and release of endothelin, which is a potent vasoconstrictor

b. **Primary hemostasis—formation of the platelet plug:**
   ○ **Endothelial injury** exposes highly thrombogenic **sub-endothelial** extracellular matrix (ECM) which leads to platelet adherence and activation.
   ○ Within minutes, the secreted products recruit additional platelets (aggregation) to form a **hemostatic plug.**

c. **Secondary hemostasis—deposition of fibrin:**
   ○ Tissue factor is released by endothelial cells following endothelial cell injury
   ○ Tissue factor along with factor VII initiates coagulation pathway and results in thrombin generation
   ○ **Thrombin** cleaves **fibrinogen** into **insoluble fibrin**, creating a **fibrin meshwork**
   ○ This will consolidate the initial platelet plug

d. **Clot stabilization and resorption:**
   ○ After clot is formed, clot stabilization and resorption is brought about by tissue plasminogen activator, t-PA

Q3. Define Virchow's triad. Write in detail about pathogenesis, morphology and fate of thrombus.

Ans.

Virchow's triad

Three primary abnormalities that lead to thrombus formation

○ Endothelial injury
○ Stasis or turbulent blood flow
○ Hypercoagulability of the blood

Pathogenesis

1. *Endothelial injury or dysfunction:*
   ○ **Causes:** Hypertension, turbulent blood flow, bacterial endotoxins, radiation injury, homocystinemia or hypercholesterolemia, cigarette smoke
   ○ Results in platelet activation and thrombus formation in heart and arterial circulation

2. *Alteration in normal blood flow:*
   - Normal blood flow is **laminar** (platelets and blood elements flow centrally in vessel lumen)
   - **Turbulent blood flow** leads to arterial and cardiac thrombosis by causing endothelial injury or dysfunction
   - Hyperviscosity (seen in polycythemia vera) increases the resistance for blood to flow and results in small vessel stasis
   - Deformed red cells in sickle cell anemia impede blood flow through small vessels
   - **Stasis** is a major contributor in the development of venous thrombi

3. *Hypercoagulability of blood:*
   - **Definition:** Any disorder of the blood that predisposes to thrombosis
   - Can be due to primary (genetic) or secondary (acquired) disorders
     - a. *Inherited (genetic) causes–*
       - Factor V gene mutation (called *Leiden* mutation)
       - Prothrombin gene mutation
       - Elevated levels of homocysteine contribute to arterial and venous thrombosis
       - Anti-thrombin III, protein C or proteins S deficiency
     - b. *Acquired causes–*
       - Prolonged bedrest or immobilization, myocardial infarction, atrial fibrillation
       - Tissue injury (surgery, fracture, and burn), cancer, prosthetic cardiac valves
       - Disseminated intravascular coagulation, heparin-induced thrombocytopenia
       - Anti-phospholipid antibody syndrome

Morphology of Thrombus
- Arterial or cardiac thrombi begin at the sites of turbulence or endothelial injury
- Venous thrombi occur at sites of stasis

a. *Antemortem thrombi:*
   - Shows **Lines of Zahn,** which represent pale platelet and fibrin deposits alternating with darker red cell-rich layers
   - Lines of Zahn signify that the thrombus has formed in the flowing blood
   - Are firm and focally attached

b. *Postmortem clots:*
   - Are **gelatinous** with dark red dependent portion where red cells have settled by gravity and a **yellow "chicken fat" upper portion**
   - Are **not attached** to the underlying wall

Arterial thrombi: Most favored sites include coronary, cerebral, and femoral arteries

Venous thrombosis (phlebothrombosis): Lower extremities are most commonly involved followed by upper extremities, periprostatic plexus, or the ovarian and periuterine veins

Fate of Thrombus

a. **Propagation:** Thrombi accumulate additional platelets and fibrin

b. **Embolization:** Thrombi dislodge and travel to other sites in the vasculature

c. **Dissolution:** As a result of fibrinolysis, there can be rapid shrinkage of recent thrombi

d. **Organization and recanalization:** Organized by the in-growth of endothelial cells, smooth muscle cells, and fibroblasts

Q4. Write a short note on heparin-induced thrombocytopenia.

Ans.

Heparin-induced thrombocytopenia (HIT) syndrome

○ Occurs following the administration of **unfractionated heparin**

○ **Unfractionated heparin** induces the formation of antibodies against complexes of **heparin and platelet factor 4**

○ Binding of antibodies to platelets results in their activation, aggregation, and consumption and hence **thrombocytopenia**

○ This leads to a **prothrombotic state**, even in face of heparin administration and low platelet counts

○ **Low-molecular weight heparin** preparations are at **lower risk** to induce antibody formation

Q5. Write a short note on antiphospholipid antibody syndrome.

Ans.

Antiphospholipid antibody syndrome (lupus anticoagulant syndrome)

○ Present with recurrent thrombosis, repeated miscarriages, cardiac valve vegetations and thrombocytopenia

○ Fetal loss occurs because of antibody-mediated interference with the growth and differentiation of trophoblasts, leading to a failure of placentation

○ Antibodies frequently give a false-positive serologic test for syphilis as the antigen in the standard assay is embedded in cardiolipin

Two types

A. **Primary antiphospholipid syndrome**—presence of a hypercoagulable state without any evidence of other autoimmune disorders

B. **Secondary antiphospholipid syndrome (lupus anticoagulant syndrome)**—individuals have an associated autoimmune disease, such as **SLE**

Q6. Enumerate types of embolism. Write a note on Caisson disease.

Ans.

Types of embolism

a. Pulmonary embolism

b. Systemic thromboembolism

c. Fat and marrow embolism

d. Air embolism

e. Amniotic fluid embolism

Air embolism
- >100 cc of air is required to have a clinical effect in the pulmonary circulation

Causes
- During bypass surgery
- Introduced into the **cerebral circulation** by neurosurgery in the "sitting position"
- During obstetric or laparoscopic procedures
- As a consequence of chest wall injury

Decompression sickness
- When individuals experience sudden decrease in atmospheric pressure
- Seen in **scuba** and **deep sea divers**, underwater construction workers, and individuals in unpressurized aircraft in rapid ascent
- During deep sea dive, when air is breathed at high pressure, increased amounts of gas (**nitrogen**) are dissolved in the blood and tissues
- When the driver ascends (**depressurizes**) **too rapidly**, nitrogen comes out of solution in the tissues and the blood resulting in damage.

Caisson disease
- **Chronic form** of **decompression sickness**
- **Ischemic necrosis**–seen in **femoral heads, tibia, and humeri** due to persistence of gas emboli in the skeletal system

Q7. Write a short note on fat embolism.

Ans.

Fat embolism
- Occurs in 90% of individuals with **severe skeletal injuries**

Fat embolism syndrome
- Symptomatic patients of fat embolism
- Characterized by **pulmonary insufficiency, neurologic symptoms, anemia, and thrombocytopenia**
- Fatal in 5% to 15% of cases

Clinical features
- Sudden onset of **tachypnea, dyspnea**, and **tachycardia**; irritability and restlessness, 1 to 3 days after injury
- **Diffuse petechial rash** due to rapid onset of thrombocytopenia is a diagnostic clue

Lab findings
- **Thrombocytopenia**—due to the platelet adhesion to fat globules
- Anemia can result from **red cell aggregation** and/or **hemolysis**
- **Paraffin embedding** cannot diagnose **fat** as these are **dissolved out** of the tissue preparations by the **solvents**
- **Frozen sections** and special **stains for fat** are used to diagnose **lipids**

Q8. Write a short note on amniotic fluid embolism.

Ans.
○ Major cause of maternal mortality worldwide
○ Occurs during labor and in immediate postpartum period

Clinical features
○ Sudden severe dyspnea, cyanosis, shock, followed by neurologic impairment (headache to seizures and coma)

Cause
○ Infusion of amniotic fluid or fetal tissue into the maternal circulation due to tear in placental membranes or rupture of uterine veins

Diagnosis
○ Requires the presence of squamous cells shed from fetal skin, lanugo hair, mucin derived from the fetal respiratory or gastrointestinal tract in the maternal pulmonary microvasculature

Q9. Write a short note on morphology of an infarct.

Ans.
Infarcts can be red (hemorrhagic) or white (anemic):
Red (hemorrhagic) infarcts:
○ Occurs with venous occlusions (e.g. **ovary**), in loose tissues (e.g. **lung**), in tissues with **dual circulations** (e.g. **lung and small intestine**)
○ When the flow is re-established to a site of previous arterial occlusion and necrosis (e.g. following **angioplasty** of an **arterial obstruction**)

White (anemic) infarcts
○ Occurs with **arterial occlusions** in **solid organs** with **end arterial circulation** (e.g. **heart, spleen, and kidney**)

Points to remember
○ Infarcts are wedge shaped
○ Dominant histology of infarction is **ischemic coagulative necrosis** except in **central nervous system infarction**, which results in **liquefactive necrosis**
○ Most of the infarcts are ultimately replaced by **scar**

Q10. Define shock, enumerate types of shock and discuss pathogenesis and morphological changes in shock.

Ans.
Definition: Shock is defined as reduced cardiac output which impairs tissue perfusion and leads to cellular hypoxia

Types of shock
1. Cardiogenic shock:
   ○ *Causes:* Myocardial infarction, ventricular rupture, arrhythmia, cardiac tamponade, pulmonary embolism

2. Hypovolemic shock
   ○ Causes: Massive hemorrhage or fluid loss from severe burns
3. Shock associated with systemic inflammation:
   ○ Causes: Microbial infections, burns, trauma, and pancreatitis
4. Neurogenic shock
   ○ Causes: Anesthetic accident or a spinal cord injury
5. Anaphylactic shock
   ○ Causes: IgE–mediated hypersensitivity reaction

Pathogenesis of Shock

a. Inflammatory cell response

   ○ Upon activation by the microbial products, innate immune cells produce TNF, IL-1, IFN-γ, IL-12, and IL-18 → results in cytokine production and endothelial activation
   ○ Activation of complement cascade → resulting in production of anaphylotoxins (C3a C5a), chemotactic fragments (C5a) and opsonins (C3b)

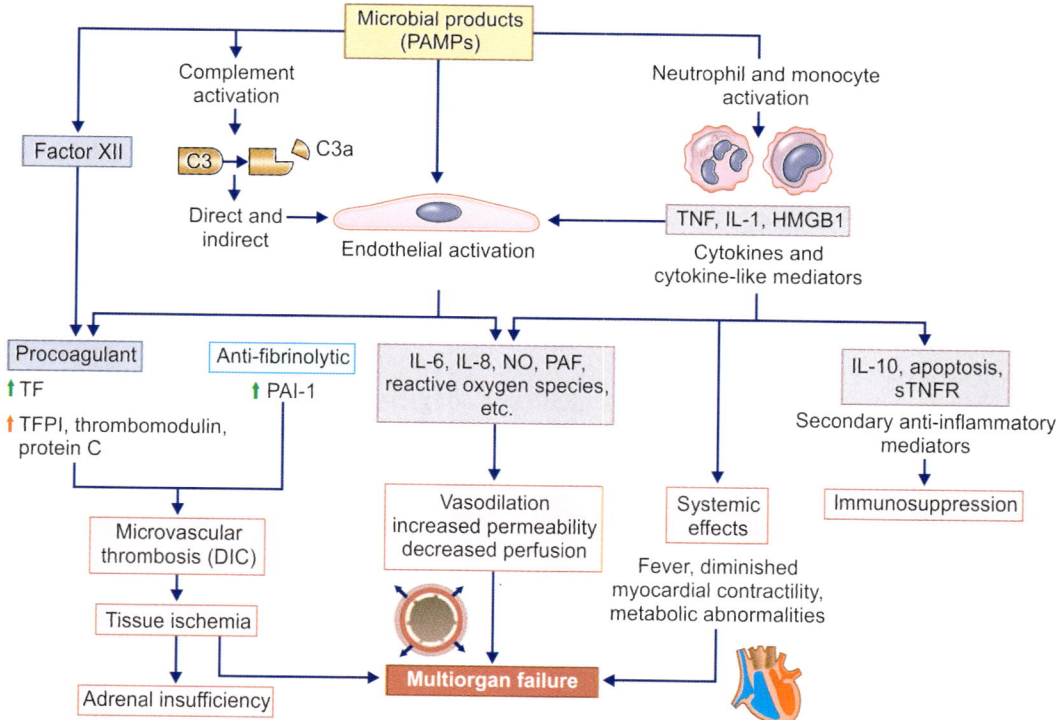

Fig. 4.1: Pathogenesis of septic shock

PAMPs: Pathogen associated molecular patterns; **HMGB1:** High mobility group box 1; **PAI–1:** Plasminogen activator inhibitor–1; **TFPI:** Tissue factor pathway inhibitor

b. Endothelial activation and injury

- ○ Activation of endothelial cells due to sepsis, leads to vascular leakage and tissue edema

c. Induction of a procoagulant state

- ○ Inflammatory cytokines favor coagulation by increasing tissue factor production by endothelial cells
- ○ Activation of widespread coagulation factors results in disseminated intravascular Coagulation (DIC) like picture
- ○ In full blown DIC, as there occurs complete utilization of coagulation factors, bleeding and hemorrhage are likely complications

d. Metabolic abnormalities

- ○ Sepsis patients exhibit insulin resistance and resultant hyperglycemia

e. Organ dysfunction

- ○ Systemic hypotension, thrombosis results in tissue hypoperfusion and resultant multiorgan failure

Morphological changes in shock

a. Adrenal gland shows cortical cell lipid depletion

b. Kidney shows acute tubular necrosis

c. Lungs show diffuse alveolar damage or shock lung

d. DIC resulting in multiple petechial hemorrhages on serosal surfaces and skin

5

Genetics

Q1. Write a note on autosomal dominant disorders with examples.

Ans.

Autosomal dominant disorders

- ○ Manifests in a heterozygous state, and one parent of an index case is usually affected
- ○ Males and females, both can be affected, and can transmit the condition
- ○ If, an affected person marries an unaffected one, every child has 50% chance of having the disease
- ○ A proportion of patients do not have affected parents (these patients have new mutations involving either the egg or the sperm, from which they were derived)
- ○ **Incomplete penetrance:** Individuals inherit the mutant gene but are phenotypically normal (BRCA-2 associated breast cancers)

Examples

System	Disorders
Nervous system	Huntington disease, neurofibromatosis, myotonic dystrophy, tuberous sclerosis
Urinary system	Polycystic kidney disease
Gastrointestinal system	Familial polyposis coli
Hematopoietic system	Hereditary spherocytosis, von Willebrand disease
Skeletal system	Marfan syndrome, Ehlers-Danlos syndrome, osteogenesis imperfecta, achondroplasia
Metabolic causes	Familial hypercholesterolemia, acute intermittent porphyria

Pedigree analysis

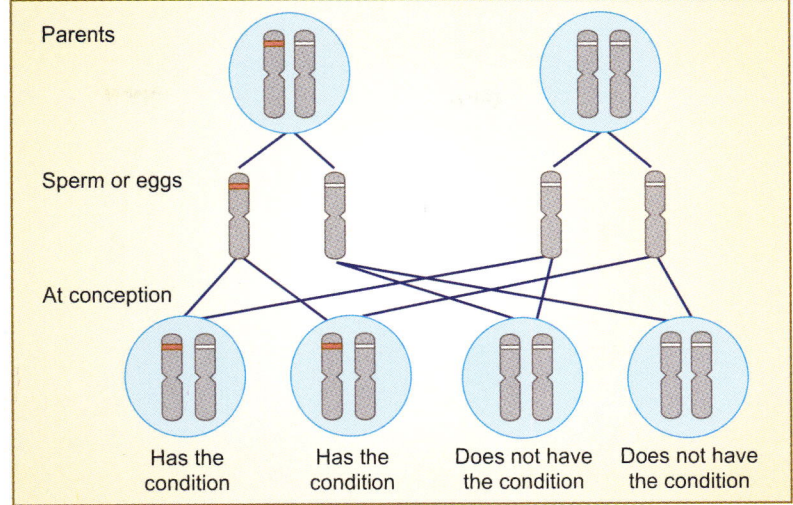

Fig. 5.1: Autosomal dominant inheritance where one parent has the condition

Q2. Write salient features of autosomal recessive disorders with examples.

Ans.

Autosomal Recessive disorders

- Occur when both alleles at a given gene locus are mutated
- Parents of an affected individual can be normal, but siblings may show the disease
- Siblings have one chance in four of having the trait (i.e. recurrence risk is 25% for each birth)
- Increased risk of transmission to siblings produced as a result of consanguineous marriages
- Complete penetrance is seen and expression of disease is more uniform

Examples

System	Disorder
Metabolic causes	Cystic fibrosis, phenylketonuria, galactosemia, homocystinuria, lysosomal storage diseases, α_1-antitrypsin deficiency, Wilson disease, hemochromatosis, glycogen storage diseases
Hematopoietic causes	Sickle cell anemia, thalassemia
Endocrine causes	Congenital adrenal hyperplasia, albinism
Skeletal causes	Ehlers-Danlos syndrome, alkaptonuria
Nervous system	Neurogenic muscular atrophies, Friedreich ataxia, spinal muscular atrophy

Pedigree analysis

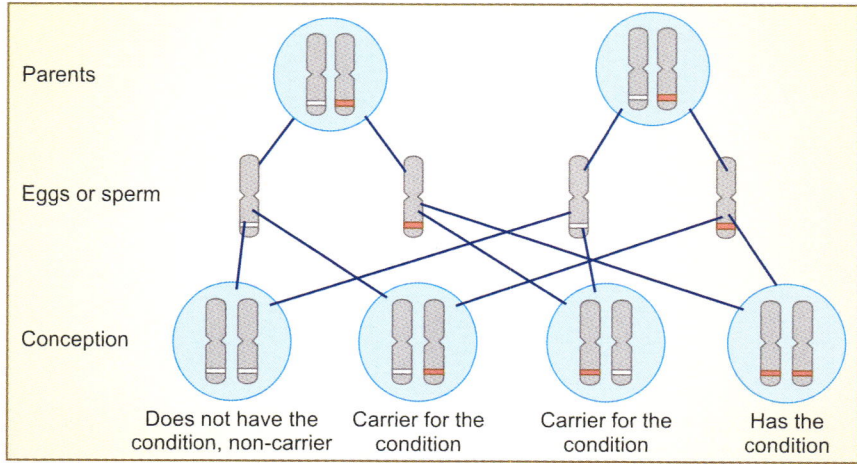

Fig. 5.2: Pedigree chart for autosomal recessive disorders

Q3. Discuss X-linked recessive disorders with examples.

Ans.

X-linked recessive disorders

○ Disorders are expressed in males

○ An affected male does not transmit the disorder to his sons, but all daughters are carriers

○ Sons of heterozygous women have, one chance in two of receiving the mutant gene

○ Because of the paired normal allele, heterozygous females are carriers (i.e., does not express full phenotypic change)

○ Heterozygous females can show the disease, if there is random inactivation of the normal X-chromosome

Examples

System	Disease
Musculoskeletal	Duchenne muscular dystrophy
Hematological	Hemophilia A and B, chronic granulomatous disease, glucose-6-phosphate dehydrogenase deficiency
Immunological	Agammaglobulinemia, Wiskott-Aldrich syndrome
Metabolic	Diabetes insipidus, Lesch-Nyhan syndrome
CNS	Fragile-X syndrome

Pedigree analysis:

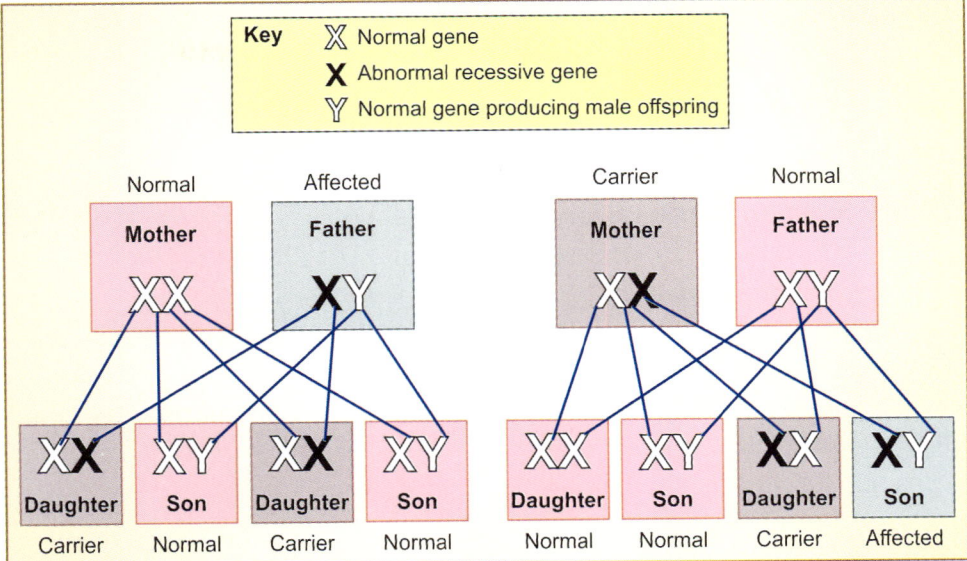

Fig. 5.3: Pedigree analysis for X-linked recessive disorders

Q4. Write a note on Marfan's syndrome.

Ans.

Marfan's syndrome

○ Shows autosomal dominant inheritance

Pathogenesis:

○ Inherited defect in the fibrillin-1 gene

○ Aorta, ligaments, and ciliary zonules that support the lens are affected (as micro fibrils are made of fibrillin)

○ Loss of microfibrils, stimulates transforming growth factor-β (TGF-β), which increases the activity of metalloproteases, resulting in loss of extracellular matrix

Morphology:

a. Skeletal abnormalities

○ Patient is tall with long extremities and long tapering fingers and toes

○ Lax joint ligaments of hands and feet, thumb can be hyperextended back to the wrist

○ Bossing of the frontal eminences and prominent supraorbital ridges

○ Kyphosis, scoliosis, rotation or slipping of the dorsal or lumbar vertebrae

○ Pectus excavatum (deeply depressed sternum) or a pigeon-breast deformity

b. *Ocular changes*
  ○ Ectopia lentis: Bilateral subluxation or dislocation (usually **outward and upward**) of the lens

c. *Cardiovascular lesions:*
  ○ Mitral valve prolapse
  ○ Aortic dissection

Q5. Write a note on familial hypercholesterolemia.

Ans.

Familial hypercholesterolemia

○ Occurs due to mutation in the gene encoding LDL receptor, involved in the transport and metabolism of cholesterol
○ Elevated plasma cholesterol levels, results in tendinous xanthomas and premature atherosclerosis

LDL metabolism

○ Liver secrete very-low density lipoproteins (VLDLs) into the bloodstream
○ Lipolysis of VLDL molecule in capillaries occurs by lipoprotein lipase, resulting in formation of intermediate-density lipoprotein (IDL)
○ VLDL molecule comprises Apo C, E, B-100, whereas IDL molecule comprises Apo E, B-100
○ IDL can be taken up by liver by LDL receptors, resulting in formation of VLDL or is converted to LDL, which is taken up by liver
○ IDL is the immediate and major source of plasma LDL
○ LDL molecule comprises Apo B-100

LDL receptor pathway and regulation of cholesterol metabolism

○ 70% of plasma LDL is cleared by liver
○ Binding of LDL to cell surface receptors, present in coated pits
○ Receptor-bound LDL are internalized by invagination to form coated vesicles
○ These coated vesicles inside the cytoplasm of the cell fuse with the lysosomes
○ In the lysosome, LDL molecule is degraded into cholesterol and ApoB-100 is degraded into amino acids
○ Free cholesterol exits through the lysosome, with the help of NPC1 and NPC2 proteins
○ LDL receptor mutations results in increased LDL levels in blood, resulting in increased deposition of cholesterol in tissues (hypercholesterolemia) and atherosclerosis

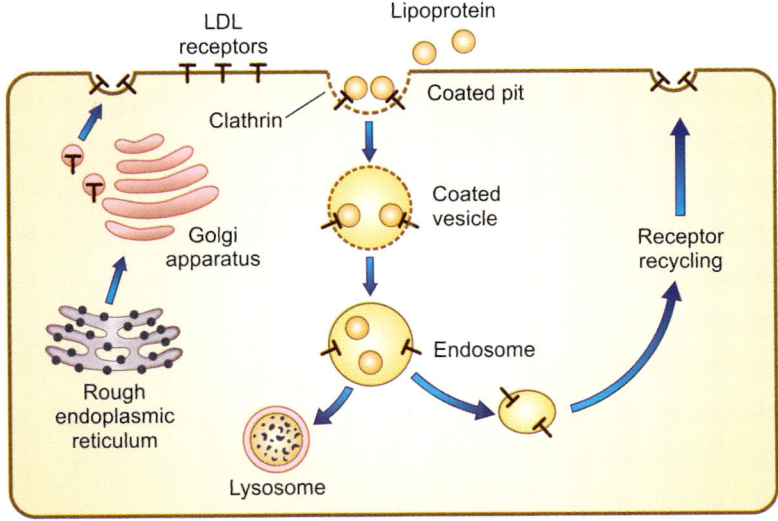

Fig. 5.4: LDL receptor pathway

Q6. Write a short note on Tay-Sachs disease.

Ans.

Tay-Sachs disease (G$_{M2}$ gangliosidosis)

○ Lysosomal storage disorder, which occurs due to deficiency of hexosaminidase, α subunit.

○ Characterized by accumulation of G$_{M2}$ ganglioside

○ Accumulation can be seen in heart, liver, spleen, however, involvement of neurons and retina dominates the clinical picture

Morphology

○ Cytoplasm of neurons shows inclusions

○ Inclusions are made up of lysosomes filled with gangliosides

○ These gangliosides are stained with oil red O or Sudan black

○ **Electron microscopy:** cytoplasmic inclusions are visualized as whorled configurations within the lysosomes

○ **Cherry-red spot** appears in the macula

Q7. Write a short note on Niemann-Pick disease.

Ans.

Niemann-Pick disease type A and B

○ Lysosomal accumulation of sphingomyelin due to an inherited deficiency of sphingomyelinase

Types

○ **Type A** (severe infantile form): Patient presents with CNS manifestations, resulting in death within first 3 years of life.
○ **Type B** patients have organomegaly, without CNS involvement

Morphology

○ Affected cells appear enlarged due to the distention of lysosomes with sphingomyelin
○ **Electron microscopy (EM)—"zebra" bodies:** Cytoplasmic bodies resembling concentric lamellated myelin figures in lysosomes
○ Numerous foamy vacuoles in the cytoplasm, which can be demonstrated by frozen section
○ Spleen: Massive splenomegaly
○ Lymphadenopathy

Niemann-Pick disease type C

○ Due to mutations in the gene NPC1 and NPC2
○ **NPC gene:** It is responsible for transport of free cholesterol from the lysosomes to the cytoplasm
○ Child presents as ataxia, dystonia, dysarthria

Q8. Write a short note on Gaucher's disease.

Ans.

Gaucher's disease

○ Autosomal recessive disorder
○ Most common lysosomal storage disorder
○ Occurs due to mutations in the gene encoding the enzyme **glucocerebrosidase**
○ Resulting in accumulation of **glucocerebroside** in macrophages
○ Thus resulting in activation of macrophages, and secretion of IL-1, IL-6, and tumor necrosis factor (TNF)

Three subtypes

○ Type I, or chronic non-neuronopathic form, in which glucocerebroside accumulates in the spleen and skeletal system
○ Type II, or acute neuronopathic Gaucher disease, death occurs at early age
○ Type III, intermediate between types I and II

Morphology

○ Massive accumulation of glucocerebrosides within the phagocytic cells throughout the body (Gaucher cells)
○ Gaucher cells are found in spleen, liver, bone marrow, lymph nodes, tonsils, thymus, and Peyer patches
○ Gaucher cells have fibrillary cytoplasm, resembling crumpled tissue paper, with a dark eccentrically placed nuclei
○ Gaucher cells show **periodic acid–Schiff** stain positivity
○ **Electron microscopy:** Fibrillary cytoplasm shows lysosomes, containing the stored lipid in the stacks of bilayers.

Diagnosis
- By measuring glucocerebrosidase activity in the peripheral blood leukocytes or in extracts of cultured skin fibroblasts

Treatment
- Replacement therapy with recombinant enzymes
- Allogeneic hematopoietic stem cell transplantation can be curative

Q9. What is principle of Karyotyping? Enumerate the stains used in the technique.

Ans.

Karyotyping
- **Definition:** Defined as the study of chromosomes
- Chromosomes are examined by arresting the dividing cells in metaphase with mitotic spindle inhibitors
- **Metaphase spread:** Individual chromosomes take the form of two chromatids connected at the centromere
- Karyotype is obtained by arranging each pair of autosomes according to their length (in decreasing order), followed by sex chromosomes
- **G banding:** Giemsa stain is used for identification of individual chromosomes on the basis of their alternative light and dark areas

Other staining patterns
- Q-Quinacrine banding demonstrates bands along chromosome
- C-banding (constitutive) demonstrates heterochromatin (chromosome material with increased density than normal)

Normal karyotyping

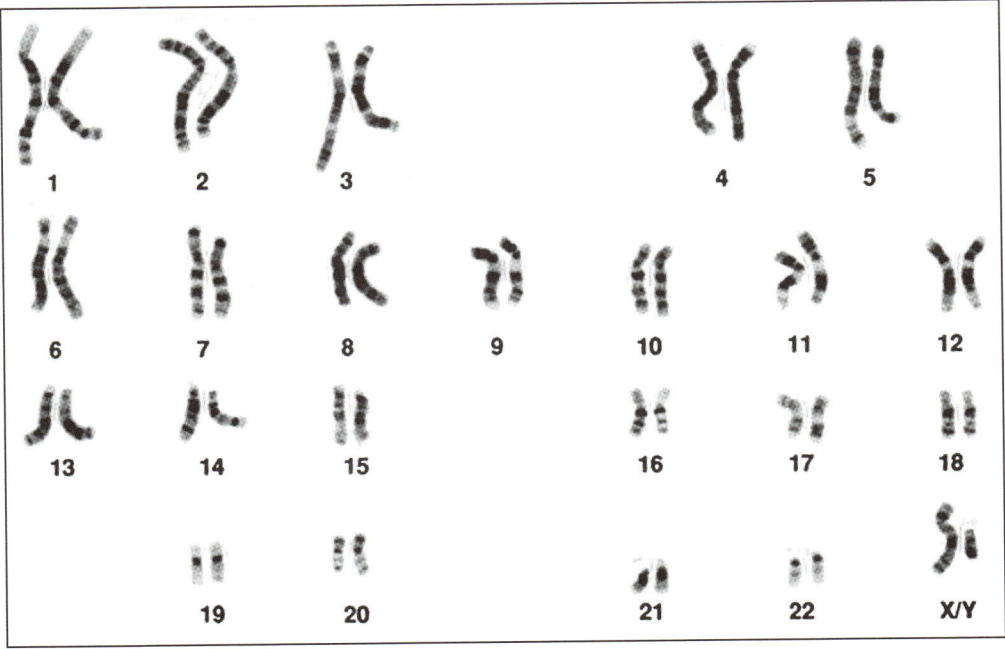

Fig. 5.5: Normal karyotyping

Q10. Enumerate different types of chromosomal rearrangements.

Ans.

Chromosomal rearrangements

- **Deletion:** Refers to loss of a portion of a chromosome, which can be interstitial or terminal
- **Ring chromosome:** Special form of deletion, which is produced when break occurs at both ends of chromosome with fusion of the damaged ends
- **Inversion:** Rearrangement that involves two breaks within a single chromosome with reincorporation of the inverted, intervening segment
- **Iso-chromosome:** When one arm of a chromosome is lost and the remaining arm is duplicated, resulting in a chromosome consisting of two short arms only or of two long arms. Most commonly seen in long arm of the X and is designated *i(X)(q10)*
- **Balanced translocation:** Segment of one chromosome is transferred to another
- **Robertsonian translocation:** Breaks occur close to the centromeres of each chromosome. Transfer of the segments then leads to one very large chromosome and one extremely small one (which is lost)

Q11. Write a short note on trisomy 21.

Ans.

Trisomy 21 (Down syndrome)

- Most common chromosomal disorder and major cause of mental retardation
- 95% of affected individuals have 47 chromosomes
- Maternal age has a strong influence on the incidence of trisomy 21

Causes

- Most common cause is **meiotic non-disjunction**, of chromosome 21, seen in **ovum**
- Robertsonian translocation of long arm of chromosome 21 to another acrocentric chromosome (e.g. 22 or 14)
- **Mosaicism:** Mixture of cells with 46 or 47 chromosomes

Clinical features

- **Most common congenital heart defect seen:** Endocardial cushion defects
- Children have increased risk of developing acute leukemia (acute megakaryoblastic leukemia being most common)
- Individuals more than 40 years develop Alzheimer disease
- Patients are prone for serious infections

Q12. Write a short note on Klinefelter syndrome.

Ans.

Klinefelter syndrome

- Common cause of hypogonadism in males
- Manifests after puberty, patients have **47, XXY karyotype** which results from **non-disjunction** during meiotic division

Clinical features

○ Eunuchoid body habitus with abnormally long legs

○ Small atrophic testes, lack of secondary male characteristics, gynecomastia

○ Mean IQ is lower than normal, but mental retardation is not seen

○ Increased incidence of type 2 diabetes and metabolic syndrome

○ Mitral valve prolapse is commonly seen in adults

○ Elevated FSH levels, with reduced testosterone levels

○ Increased risk for breast cancer, extra-gonadal germ cell tumors and autoimmune diseases like SLE

○ An important genetic cause of reduced spermatogenesis and male infertility

Q13. Write a short note on Turner's syndrome.

Ans.

Turner's syndrome

○ Results from complete or partial monosomy of the X chromosome

○ Characterized by hypogonadism in phenotypic females

○ Most common sex chromosome abnormality in females

○ Most common structural abnormality of X chromosome includes 45, X

Clinical features

In infants

○ Presents with edema of the dorsum of the hand and foot due to lymph stasis

○ Swelling of the nape of the neck (cystic hygroma)

○ Congenital heart disease—pre-ductal coarctation of the aorta and bicuspid aortic valve

In adults

○ Short stature, webbing of neck, low posterior hairline

○ Streak gonads, primary infertility (most common cause)

○ Broad chest, widely separated nipples and pigmented nevi

Note

○ **Short stature homeobox (SHOX)** gene at **Xp22.33** is responsible for short stature

Q14. Discuss Fragile-X syndrome.

Ans.

Fragile-X syndrome

○ Second most common genetic cause of mental retardation, after Down syndrome

○ Caused by mutation in familial mental retardation-1 (FMR-1) gene, located on chromosome Xq27.3

○ There appears a constriction or discontinuity of staining in the long arm of X chromosome, and it appears that chromosome is "broken", hence it was named fragile site

Salient features

○ **Anticipation:** Clinical features of fragile X syndrome worsen with each successive generation

○ **FMR1 gene** located on chromosome Xq27.3, in normal population encodes CGG trinucleotide repeats, number varying from 6-55

○ **Premutations:** Normal transmitting males and carrier females carry 55 to 200 CGG repeats

○ **Full mutations:** Affected individuals show 200 to 4000 CGG repeats

Pedigree analysis

○ In the first generation all sons are normal and all females are carriers

○ During oogenesis in the carrier female, premutation expands to full mutation; hence, in the next generation all males who inherit the X with full mutation are affected

○ Carrier male, transmit the repeats, with small number of changes

○ When a carrier female, transmits the repeats, dramatic amplification of the CGG repeats are seen, leading to mental retardation in male offspring and 50% female offspring

○ Hence, pre-mutations are converted to mutations by triple nucleotide repeat amplification, which occurs during the process of oogenesis

Clinical features

○ Affected males have long face with large mandible, large everted ears, and large testicles (macro-orchidism, most distinctive feature)

○ Hyperextensible joints, high-arched palate, and mitral valve prolapse

Q15. Write a note on mitochondrial inheritance.

Ans.

Mitochondrial genes mutations

○ Mitochondrial DNA is maternally inherited, as ova contains numerous mitochondria within its cytoplasm

○ Mothers transmit the disease to their sons and daughters, and sons do not transmit the disease to their progeny

○ As mtDNA encodes enzymes involved in oxidative phosphorylation, mutations affecting these genes exert their deleterious effects primarily on the organs most dependent on oxidative phosphorylation such as the central nervous system, skeletal muscle, cardiac muscle, liver, and kidneys

○ For example, CPEO (Chronic progressive external ophthalmoplegia), KSS (Kearns-Sayre syndrome), Pearson syndrome, Leigh syndrome, NARP (neurogenic weakness with ataxia and retinitis pigmentosa), MELAS (mitochondrial encephalopathy with lactic acidosis and stroke-like episodes), MERRF (myoclonic epilepsy with ragged red fibres), LHON (Leber hereditary optic neuropathy)

Q16. Write a note on genomic imprinting with examples.

Ans.

Genomic imprinting
○ Every individual inherit two copies of each autosomal gene, from mother (maternal chromosome) and from father (paternal chromosome)
○ Imprinting selectively inactivates either the maternal or paternal allele
○ Maternal imprinting refers to silencing of the maternal allele
○ Paternal imprinting refers to silencing of paternal allele
○ Imprinting occurs in the ovum or the sperm, before fertilization, and is transmitted to all somatic cells through mitosis

a. Prader-Willi syndrome
○ Occurs due to deletion of paternally derived chromosome 15
○ Characterized by mental retardation, short stature, hypotonia, profound hyperphagia, obesity, small hands and feet, and hypogonadism

b. Angelman syndrome
○ Occurs due to deletion of maternally derived chromosome 15
○ Characterized by mental retardation, ataxic gait, seizures, and inappropriate laughter
○ Because of their laughter and ataxia they have been referred to as "happy puppets"

Q17. Write a short note on Fluorescent *in situ* hybridization.

Ans.

Fluorescence in situ hybridization (FISH)
○ Uses DNA probes that recognize sequences specific to particular chromosomal regions

Samples on which FISH can be performed
○ Prenatal samples, peripheral blood cells, touch preparations from cancer biopsies

Uses
○ To detect aneuploidy, microdeletions, translocations, gene amplification (e.g., HER2 in breast cancer or NMYC amplification in neuroblastomas)
○ Determination of treatment efficacy, e.g. in BCR-ABL positive CML
○ Definitive diagnosis of HPV

6

Immunity

Q1. Define innate immunity. What are the components of innate immunity?

Ans.

○ **Definition:** Innate immunity refers to the mechanisms that are ready to react to infections even before they occur

Components of innate immunity include:

○ **Epithelial barriers:** Epithelia of the skin, gastrointestinal and respiratory tracts, which prevent the entry of microbe

○ **Monocyte and neutrophils:** Are phagocytes in the blood that can be recruited to the site of infection

○ **Dendritic cells:** Are antigen presenting cells and display the microbial peptides to T-lymphocytes

○ **Natural killer cells:** Protects against viruses

○ Mast cells and proteins of complement system

Q2. Write a short note on toll-like receptors.

Ans.

Toll-like receptors (TLRs)

○ Act as cellular receptor for microbes in innate immunity

○ Are present in the plasma membrane and endosomal vesicles of the cell

○ Microbe when comes in contact with a cell, is recognized by these toll-like receptors

○ Following the microbe recognition, toll-like receptors send signals which result in activation of **NF-κB** and **interferon regulatory factors**

○ **NF-κB** stimulates the synthesis and secretion of cytokines, which recruits neutrophils

○ **Interferon regulatory factors** (IRFs) produces antiviral cytokines, like type I interferon

○ Both of these result in control of microbial infection

Q3. Write a short note on T cell receptor complex.

Ans.

○ T-lymphocytes are classified into helper T lymphocytes, cytotoxic T lymphocytes (CTLs) and regulatory T lymphocytes

T cell receptor complex comprises:

- ○ TCR heterodimer consists of α and β chain, recognizes antigen, expressed by MHC molecule on antigen presenting cells (APCs)
- ○ CD3 complex and ζ chains of T cell receptor complex, initiate the activating signals
- ○ Other than CD4, T cells also express CD8 molecules
- ○ **CD4+ T cells:** In response to the antigen, it stimulates cytokine production
- ○ **CD8+ T cells:** It functions as cytotoxic (killer) T cells
- ○ **Function:** T cell recognizes specific cell-bound antigen by means of an antigen-specific TCR

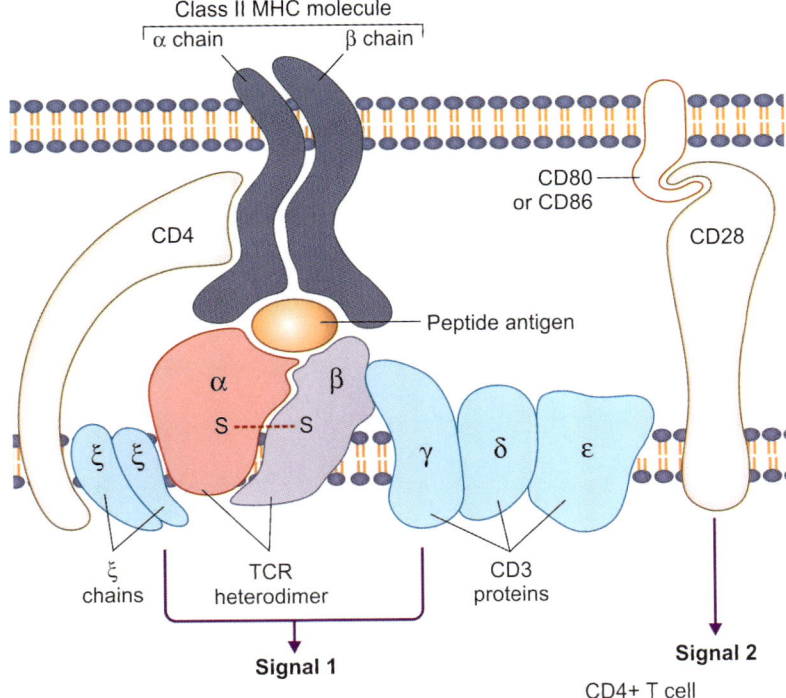

Fig. 6.1: Antigen-presenting cell

Q4. Write briefly on natural killer cells.

Ans.

Natural killer cells

- ○ Also called large granular lymphocytes, as they contain abundant azurophilic granules
- ○ They can kill infected cells and tumor cells, without prior exposure to activation by these microbes/tumors
- ○ They act as an early line of defense against viral infections and tumors
- ○ **CD16** and **CD56** are used to identify NK cells

○ **Antibody-dependent cell-mediated cytotoxicity:** CD16 on NK cell is an Fc receptor for IgG, and confers NK cells the ability to lyse IgG-coated target cells

○ NK cells secrete **interferon-γ (IFN-γ)**, which activates macrophages to destroy ingested microbes

Q5. Write a note on major histocompatibility complex and its structure.

Ans.

Major histocompatibility complex (MHC)

○ Display peptide fragments of proteins for recognition by T cells (antigen specific)

○ Also called human leukocyte antigens (HLA)

○ Genes encoding HLA are located on chromosome 6

Class I MHC molecules

○ Are expressed on all nucleated cells and platelets

○ They are heterodimers consisting of "α or heavy chain" linked to a smaller peptide chain called "β_2-microglobulin"

○ α chains are encoded by three genes: HLA-A, HLA-B, and HLA-C

○ α chain is divided into three domains: α_1, α_2, and α_3

○ α_1 and α_2 domains form a cleft, or groove, where peptides bind

○ α_3 domain has a binding site for CD8+ T cells (cytotoxic T-lymphocytes)

○ As CD8+ T cells recognize the peptides presented by class I MHC molecules, CD8+ T cells are class I MHC restricted

Class II MHC molecules

○ Encoded in a region called HLA-D, which has three sub-regions: HLA-DP, HLA-DQ, and HLA-DR

○ They are heterodimer composed of α chain and β chain, and both have two domains designated α_1 and α_2, and β_1 and β_2

○ Peptide-binding cleft formed by an interaction of the α_1 and β_1 domains

○ β_2 domain has a binding site for CD4

○ As CD4+ T cells recognize peptides/antigens presented by class II MHC molecules, CD4+ T cells are class II MHC restricted

Class III MHC molecules

○ Encodes complement components and the cytokines (TNF and lymphotoxin)

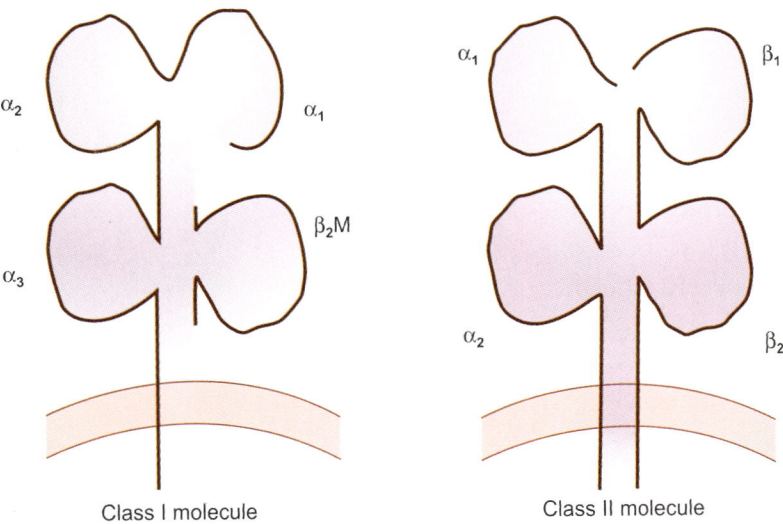

Class I molecule   Class II molecule

Fig. 6.2: MHC molecules

Q6. Define hypersensitivity. Discuss in detail about type I hypersensitivity reactions.

Ans.

○ **Hypersensitivity**: Implies an excessive or harmful reaction to antigen

Immediate (type I) hypersensitivity

○ **Definition:** Rapid immunologic reaction, which occurs within minutes, after the antigen combines to the antibody bound to the mast cells, seen in individuals, who are previously sensitized to the antigen

Two well-defined phases

a. *Immediate reaction*
  ○ Occurs within minutes after exposure to an allergen and subsides within a few hours
  ○ Characterized by vasodilatation, vascular leakage and smooth muscle spasm

b. *Late phase reaction*
  ○ Occurs 2–24 hours later
  ○ It is characterized by infiltration of tissues with eosinophils, neutrophils, basophils, monocytes and CD4+ T cells with resultant mucosal epithelial cell damage
  ○ Helper T cells are classified into TH1 cells, TH2 cells and TH17 cells
  ○ TH2 cells play a role in type I hypersensitivity reactions

Role of TH2 cells

○ Antigen when enters the body is captured by dendritic cells, which present it to naïve CD4 + T cells

○ Naïve CD4+ T cells, in response to the antigen, release IL-4 and differentiates into TH2 cells

○ TH2 cells produce cytokines IL-4, IL-5, and IL-13

○ IL-4 acts on B cells to stimulate IgE production, which binds to the mast cells (mast cells express FcεRI, specific for Fc portion of IgE)

○ IgE-coated mast cells, if exposed to similar antigen, result in mast cell activation and there occurs release of mediators, which bring about the clinical expression of immediate hypersensitivity reactions

Mediators of type I hypersensitivity reactions:

1. **Preformed mediators:** Present within mast cell granules, and are divided into 3 categories:

   a. **Vasoactive amines:** Like histamine which brings about smooth muscle contraction, increased vascular permeability and increased mucus secretion

   b. **Enzymes:** Proteases

   c. **Proteoglycans:** Heparin, chondroitin sulfate

2. **Lipid Mediators:**

   ○ Phospholipase A2 in mast cells convert membrane phospholipids to arachidonic acid

   a. Arachidonic acid metabolites

   ○ **Leukotrienes B4, C4, D4:**

   – LTC4 and D4 are most potent vasoactive agents, increases vascular permeability, bronchial smooth muscle contraction

   – LTB4 is chemotactic for neutrophils, eosinophils, and monocytes

   ○ **Prostaglandin D2:** Results in bronchospasm and increased mucus secretion

   b. Platelet-activating factor (PAF):

   ○ Platelet aggregation, release of histamine, bronchospasm, increased vascular permeability, and vasodilation

3. **Cytokines:**

   ○ TNF, IL-1, and chemokines: Leukocyte recruitment (in late phase reaction)

   ○ IL-4: Amplifies TH2 response

Examples of type I hypersensitivity reactions: Anaphylaxis, bronchial asthma, allergic rhinitis, hay fever, food allergies

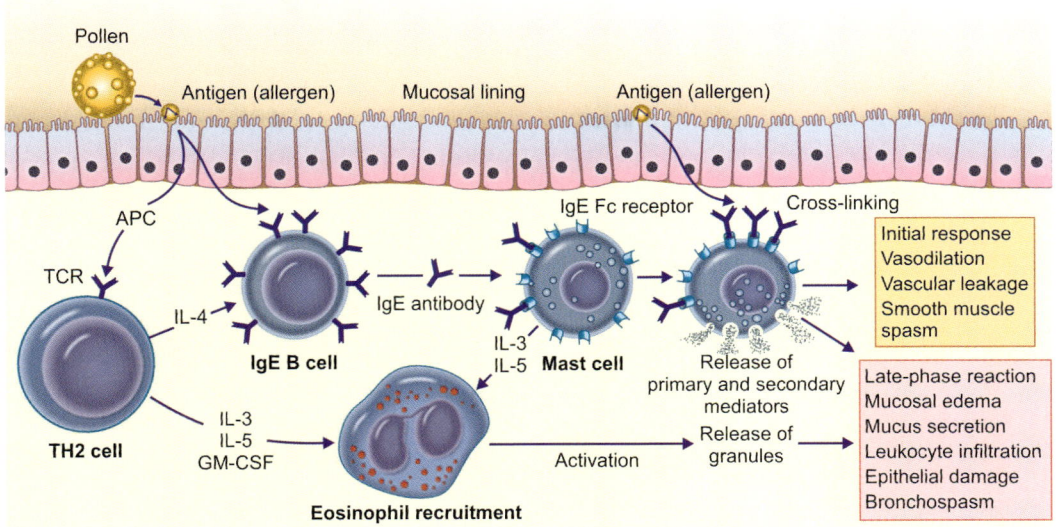

Fig. 6.3: Events in type I hypersensitivity reactions

Q7. Discuss in detail Type II Hypersensitivity reactions with examples.

Ans.

Antibody-mediated (type II) hypersensitivity

○ Caused by antibodies that react with antigens present on the cell surface or in the extracellular matrix

Antibody-mediated mechanisms

a. *Opsonization and phagocytosis:*

○ IgM or IgG antibodies on the cell surface, activates the complement system by classical pathway, resulting in deposition of C3b or C4b on cell surface, which is recognized by phagocytes, resulting in phagocytosis of the opsonized cells

○ Cells opsonized by IgG antibodies are recognized by phagocyte Fc receptors, which are specific for the Fc portions of IgG subclasses

○ For example: Transfusion reactions, erythroblastosis fetalis, autoimmune hemolytic anemia, agranulocytosis, thrombocytopenia

b. *Inflammation*

○ Antibodies deposited on the basement membrane stimulates the complement system and results in activation of complement by products like C5a and C3a

○ C5a and C3a result in activation of neutrophils, monocytes and increased vascular permeability

○ Activated leucocytes release mediators which damage basement membrane, collagen, elastin, and cartilage

c. *Cellular dysfunction*

○ Antibodies are formed against cell surface receptors, which impair or dysregulate its function, e.g.

a. Myasthenia gravis, antibodies are formed against ACh receptor in the motor end plate of skeletal muscles, blocking neuromuscular transmission and muscle weakness

b. Graves' disease, antibodies against the thyroid-stimulating hormone receptor on thyroid epithelial cells stimulate the cells, resulting in hyperthyroidism

Examples of type II hypersensitivity reactions

○ Autoimmune hemolytic anemia, autoimmune idiopathic thrombocytopenic purpura, pemphigus vulgaris, vasculitis caused by ANCA, Goodpasture syndrome, acute rheumatic fever, myasthenia gravis, Graves' disease, insulin resistant diabetes

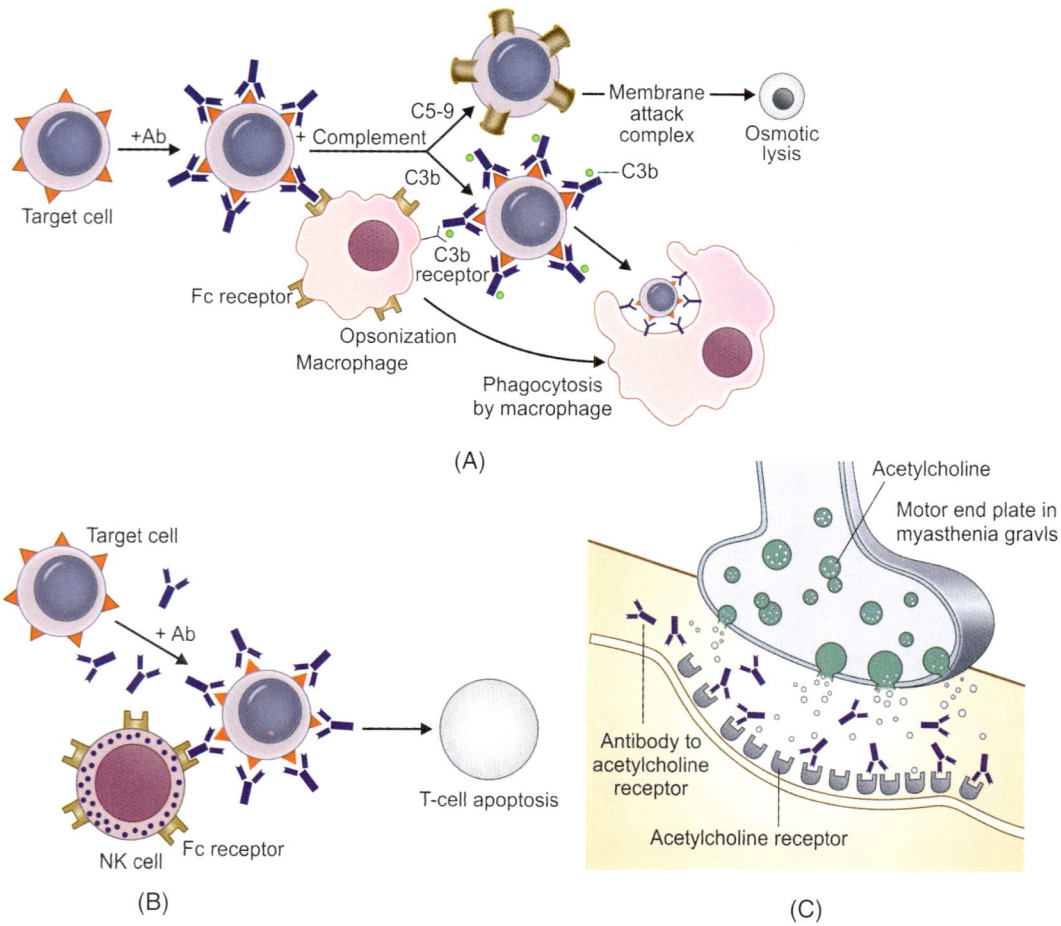

Fig. 6.4: (A) Complement mediated; (B) Antibody dependent cell-mediated cytotoxicity (ADCC); (C) Antireceptor antibodies

Q8. Write a short note on type III hypersensitivity reactions.

Ans.

Immune complex-mediated (type III) hypersensitivity
- Antigen–antibody complex gets deposited in the vessel wall and produces tissue damage by eliciting inflammation
- Antigen can be exogenous or endogenous (autoimmunity)
- Can be systemic (immune complexes in circulation) or can involve kidney, joints and small blood vessels

Two types
1. *Systemic immune complex disease*
   - Acute serum sickness is the prototype

   Pathogenesis: Divided into three phases:
   a. Formation of antigen–antibody complexes in the circulation
   b. Deposition of immune complexes: Most commonly affects glomeruli and joints
   c. Inflammation and tissue injury by immune complexes

2. *Local immune complex disease (Arthus reaction)*
   - Results from acute immune complex vasculitis, elicited in the skin
   - Can be produced experimentally by intra-cutaneous injection of an antigen in a previously immunized animal

Examples of type III hypersensitivity reaction
- SLE, post streptococcal glomerulonephritis, polyarteritis nodosa, reactive arthritis, serum sickness and Arthus reaction

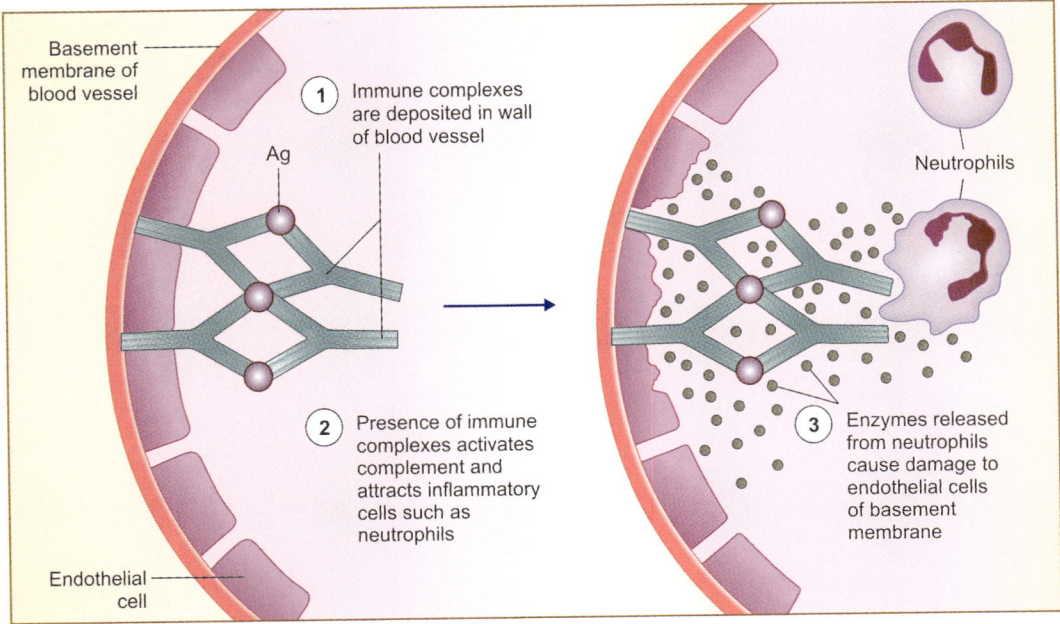

Fig. 6.5: Immune complexes mediated blood vessel wall damage

Q9. Discuss type IV hypersensitivity reaction with examples.

Ans.

T cell-mediated (type IV) hypersensitivity: Can be induced by CD4+ T cells and CD8+ T cells

1. CD4+ T cell-mediated inflammation

- Cytokines produced by T cells induce inflammation
- Presents as **delayed-type hypersensitivity (DTH)**

Example of DTH

a. **Tuberculin reaction:**
   - Produced by intra-cutaneous injection of purified protein derivative (PPD)/ tuberculin, in previously sensitized individual, reddening and in duration of the site appears in 8–12 hours, reach a peak in 24–72 hours and slowly subside

b. **Contact dermatitis**

c. Rheumatoid arthritis, multiple sclerosis, inflammatory bowel disease

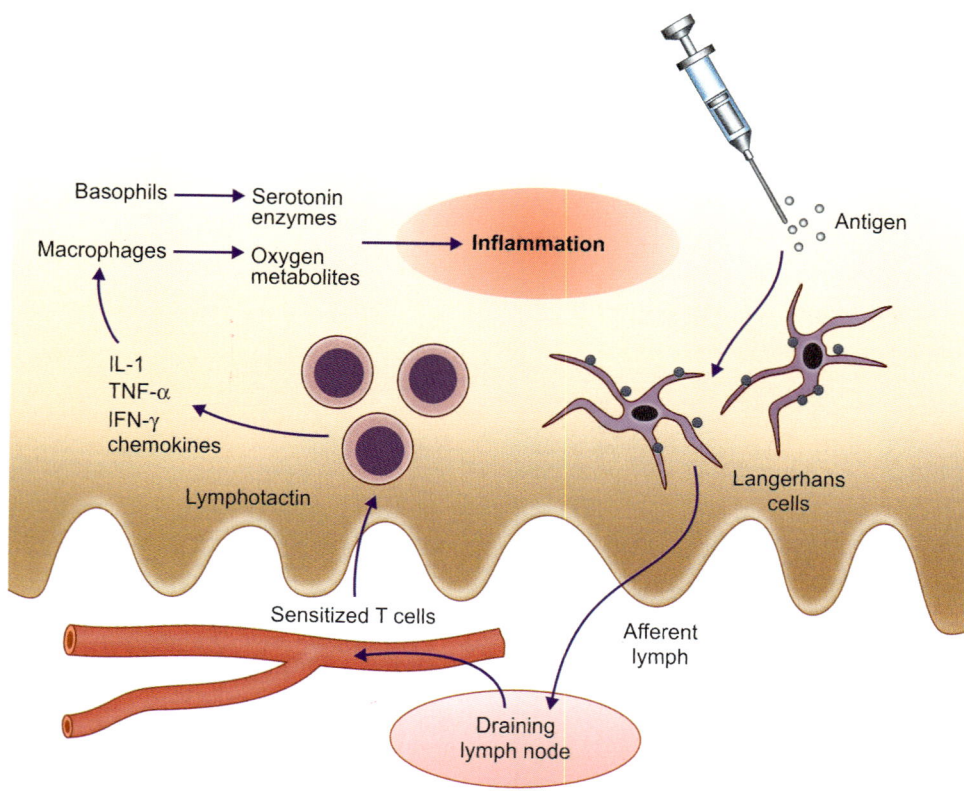

Fig. 6.6: Tuberculin reaction

2. CD8+ T cell-mediated cytotoxicity

- CD8+ cytotoxic T-lmphocytes (CTLs) kill antigen-expressing target cells
- **Examples:** Seen in type I DM, graft rejection and reactions against viruses

Q10. Write a note on mechanism of autoimmune diseases.

Ans.

First we need to understand the concept of tolerance!
- Tolerance means unresponsiveness to self-antigens, which is a fundamental property of the immune system
- In autoimmune diseases, there is breakdown of tolerance

Mechanisms of self-tolerance: Two types
- **Central tolerance:** In thymus and bone marrow, immature lymphocytes that recognize self-antigens are killed by apoptosis
- **Peripheral tolerance:** Cells that escape central organs, come into the peripheral blood and are inactivated in peripheral lymphoid system

1. **Central tolerance**
   - Immature T and B lymphocytes, during their maturation in thymus (T cells) and bone marrow (B cells), recognize self-antigens and kill them by:
     a. **Negative selection/ deletion:** In thymus, immature lymphocytes encounter the antigen → cells die of apoptosis
     b. **Receptor editing:** B cells recognize self-antigens in the bone marrow, and begin to express new antigen receptors, not specific for self-antigens

2. **Peripheral tolerance**
   - Mechanisms that silence potentially auto-reactive T and B cells in peripheral tissues
     a. **Anergy**
        - Functional inactivation of lymphocytes, that recognize self-antigens
     b. **Suppression by regulatory T cells**
        - **Regulatory T cells** function to prevent immune reactions against self-antigens
     c. **Deletion by apoptosis**
        - T cells that recognize self-antigens may die by apoptosis, which can occur due to activation of pro-apoptotic molecule **Bim** or activation-induced death of CD4+ T cells and B cells by Fas-Fas ligand system

Mechanisms/pathogenesis of autoimmune diseases

a. *Role of susceptibility genes*
   - Most autoimmune diseases are complex multigenic disorders
   - **Examples:** HLA-B27 association with ankylosing spondylitis, non-MHC genes like polymorphisms in PTNP22 associated with type I DM, rheumatoid arthritis, polymorphisms in NOD2 associated with Crohn disease

b. *Role of Infections*
   - Infection induces co-stimulators on antigen presenting cells, which result in activation of T cells, resulting in tissue destruction
   - **Molecular mimicry:** Microbes express antigens that resemble self-antigen, which results in activation of self-reactive lymphocytes, e.g. rheumatic heart disease

Q11. Enumerate revised criteria for classification of systemic lupus erythematosus (SLE).

Ans.

Revised criteria for classification of systemic lupus erythematosus

1. Malar rash: Erythema over malar eminences
2. Discoid rash: Erythematous raised patches with scaling and plugging
3. Photosensitivity: Rash due to sunlight
4. Oral ulcers: Oral or nasopharyngeal ulceration
5. Arthritis: Non-erosive arthritis involving two or more peripheral joints
6. Serositis: Pleuritis or pericarditis
7. Renal disorder: Persistent proteinuria > 0.5 gm% or cellular casts
8. Neurologic disorder: Seizures, psychosis
9. Hematological disorder: Hemolytic anemia with reticulocytosis or leucopenia or lymphopenia or thrombocytopenia
10. Immunologic disorder:
    ○ Anti-DNA antibody or anti-Sm antibody or positive finding of antiphospholipid antibody syndrome
11. Antinuclear antibody: Abnormal titer of ANA by immunofluorescence

Note: A person is said to have SLE if any four or more of the 11 criteria are present.

Q12. Discuss antibodies specific for SLE and pathogenesis of the disease.

Ans.

Antinuclear antibodies (ANAs) in SLE are directed against nuclear antigens and grouped into 4 categories:

a. Antibodies to DNA

b. Antibodies to histone

c. Antibodies to non-histone proteins bound to RNA

d. Antibodies to nucleolar antigens

Etiology and pathogenesis of SLE

a. *Genetic factors*
   ○ HLA-DQ locus alleles are responsible for production of anti-double stranded DNA, anti-Sm, and antiphospholipid antibodies
   ○ Lupus patients have inherited deficiencies of C2, C4, or C1q which impairs removal of circulating immune complexes by mononuclear phagocyte system and thus favoring tissue deposition

b. *Immunologic factors*
   ○ Nuclear DNA and RNA in antigen–antibody complexes stimulate B-lymphocytes resulting in increased production of anti-nuclear antibodies

c. *Environmental factors*
  ○ Exposure to ultraviolet (UV) light, induces apoptosis in cells, these apoptotic cell becomes immunogenic and exacerbates the disease
  ○ UV light stimulates keratinocytes, which release IL-1 and promotes inflammation
  ○ Drugs: Hydralazine, procainamide, D-penicillamine can induce an SLE-like response

Q13. Discuss the renal morphology in SLE.

Ans.

Lupus nephritis
○ Glomerular lesions occur due to immune complex deposition

Six patterns of glomerular disease are seen in SLE

a. *Minimal mesangial lupus nephritis (class I)*
  ○ Least common, immune complex deposition in the mesangium, confirmed by immunoflourescence microscopy (IF) and EM (electron microscopy)

b. *Mesangial proliferative lupus nephritis (class II)*
  ○ Mesangial cell proliferation and accumulation of mesangial matrix

c. *Focal lupus nephritis (class III):*
  ○ Involvement of fewer than 50% of all glomeruli
  ○ Lesions may be segmental (affecting only a portion of the glomerulus) or global (involving the entire glomerulus)
  ○ Glomeruli show swelling and proliferation of endothelial and mesangial cells with leukocyte accumulation, capillary necrosis, and hyaline thrombi

d. *Diffuse lupus nephritis (class IV)*
  ○ Most common and severe form of lupus nephritis
  ○ Half or more of the glomeruli are affected
  ○ Involved glomeruli show proliferation of endothelial, mesangial and epithelial cells
  ○ **Wire loop structures:** Sub-endothelial immune complex deposits leading to circumferential thickening of the capillary wall on light microscopy

e. *Membranous lupus nephritis (class V)*
  ○ Diffuse thickening of the capillary walls due to deposition of sub-epithelial immune complexes
  ○ Severe proteinuria or nephrotic syndrome

f. *Advanced sclerosing lupus nephritis (class VI)*
  ○ Sclerosis of more than 90% of the glomeruli represents end-stage renal disease

Q14. What is LE cell?

Ans.

○ Antinuclear antibodies (ANAs) are seen in SLE patients

○ ANAs cannot penetrate intact cell, but in tissues, nuclei of damaged cells react with ANA's, which now lose their chromatin pattern and become homogenous to produce **"LE bodies"** or **"hematoxylin bodies"**

○ **LE cell** is any phagocytic leukocyte (neutrophil or macrophage), that has engulfed the denatured nucleus of an injured cell

Q15. Write a note on transplant rejection.

Ans.

○ **Rejection:** Mechanism by which the recipient's immune system recognizes the graft as foreign and attacks it

Mechanism of rejection

○ **T lymphocytes** and **antibodies** produced against graft antigens react against and destroy tissue graft

a. *Lymphocyte mediated destruction*

○ T cell mediated rejection is brought about by CD4 and CD8 T cells, which recognize the graft antigens, presented by donor antigen presenting cell

b. *Antibody mediated destruction*

○ Brought about by preformed antibodies or antibodies produced due to donor antigens

Morphology

○ Rejection of kidney grafts are classified into: Hyperacute, acute, and chronic forms

Q16. Write a short note on hyper-IgM syndrome.

Ans.

Hyper-IgM syndrome

○ Patients can produce IgM antibodies, but not IgG, IgA or IgE antibodies

○ CD4+ helper T cells expresses CD40 molecule

○ Because of expression of CD40 molecule, CD4+ T cell recognizes CD40L (ligand) on B cells, macrophages and dendritic cells, resulting in activation of B-cells

○ In hyper IgM syndrome, CD40L is mutated

○ Serum of these patients contain normal or elevated levels of IgM, but no IgA or IgE and extremely low levels of IgG, although the number of B and T cells is normal

○ Presents as recurrent pyogenic infections, *Pneumocystis jiroveci* pneumonia

○ IgM antibodies react with blood cells, giving rise to autoimmune hemolytic anemia, thrombocytopenia, and neutropenia

Q17. Write a note on opportunistic infections and neoplasms in AIDS.

Ans.

AIDS: Defining opportunistic infections and neoplasms in HIV infected patients:

A. Infections

1. Protozoal and helminthic infections
- Cryptosporidiosis or isosporidiosis (enteritis)
- Pneumocystosis (pneumonia or disseminated infection)
- Toxoplasmosis (pneumonia or CNS infection)

2. Fungal infections
- Candidiasis (esophageal, tracheal, or pulmonary)
- Cryptococcosis (CNS infection)
- Coccidioidomycosis (disseminated)
- Histoplasmosis (disseminated)

3. Bacterial infections
- Mycobacteriosis (*Mycobacterium avium-intracellulare, Mycobacterium tuberculosis*)
- Nocardiosis (pneumonia, meningitis, disseminated)
- Salmonella infections, disseminated

4. Viral infections
- Cytomegalovirus (pulmonary, intestinal, retinitis, or CNS infections)
- Herpes simplex virus
- Varicella-zoster virus
- Progressive multifocal leukoencephalopathy

B. Neoplasms
- Kaposi sarcoma
- Primary lymphoma of brain
- Invasive cancer of uterine cervix

Q18. Discuss in detail the pathogenesis and classification of amyloidosis and staining characteristics of amyloid.

Ans.
- **Amyloid:** Pathologic proteinaceous substance, which on hematoxylin and eosin (H&E) stain, appears as amorphous, eosinophilic, hyaline, extracellular substance

Pathogenesis of amyloidosis:
- Results from abnormal folding of proteins, which are deposited as fibrils in extracellular tissues and disrupt normal function
- Normally, misfolded proteins are degraded intracellularly in proteasomes or extracellularly by macrophages
- In amyloidosis, these mechanisms fail and misfolded protein accumulates outside cells

Classification of Amyloidosis

Clinicopathologic category	Major fibril protein	Related precursor protein
A. Systemic (generalized) amyloidosis		
Immunocyte dyscrasias with amyloidosis (primary amyloidosis)	AL	Immunoglobulin light chains, chiefly λ type
Reactive systemic amyloidosis (secondary amyloidosis)	AA	SAA
Hemodialysis-associated amyloidosis	$A\beta_2 m$	β_2-microglobulin
B. Hereditary amyloidosis		
Familial Mediterranean fever	AA	SAA
Familial amyloidotic neuropathies	ATTR	Transthyretin
Systemic senile amyloidosis	ATTR	Transthyretin
C. Localized amyloidosis		
Senile cerebral	$A\beta$	APP
Medullary carcinoma of thyroid	A Cal	Calcitonin
Islets of Langerhans	AIAPP	Islet amyloid peptide
Isolated atrial amyloidosis	AANF	Atrial natriuretic factor

Staining pattern of amyloid
- Most common stain used is Congo red
- Congo red, under ordinary light, imparts pink or red color to amyloid
- Under polarized light, Congo red-stained amyloid shows apple-green birefringence

Q19. Write a note on pathology of spleen in amyloidosis and mention the physical properties of amyloid.

Ans.

Morphology of spleen in amyloidosis:
- Results in splenomegaly
- **Sago spleen:** Amyloid deposits are limited to the splenic follicles, producing tapioca-like granules on gross inspection
- **Lardaceous spleen:** Amyloid deposits in the walls of the splenic sinuses and in red pulp, producing large map like areas

Physical nature of amyloid
- **Electron microscopy:** Amyloid appears as continuous, non-branching fibrils with a diameter of approximately 7.5 to 10 nm
- **X-ray crystallography:** Amyloid shows characteristic cross-β-pleated sheet conformation

7

Neoplasia

Q1. Define Neoplasia.

Ans.

- **Definition (pre-molecular era):** Abnormal mass of tissue, the growth of which exceeds and is uncoordinated with that of the normal tissues and persists in the same excessive manner after cessation of the stimuli which evoked the change
- **Definition (molecular era):** Disorder of cell growth that is triggered by series of acquired mutations affecting a single cell and its clonal progeny.

Q2. Differences between benign and malignant tumors.

Ans.

Features	Benign	Malignant
Boundaries	Encapsulated or well-circumscribed	Poorly circumscribed or irregular
Surrounding tissue	Compressed	Invaded
Secondary changes, i.e. hemorrhage and necrosis	Less common	More common
Pattern	Resemble to the tissue of origin	No resemblance
Nucleo-cytoplasmic ratio	Normal	Increased
Pleomorphism	Absent	Present
Anisonucleosis	Absent	Present
Hyperchromasia	Absent	Present
Growth rate	Slow	Rapid
Metastasis	Absent	Present

Q3. Define metaplasia with examples.

Ans.

Metaplasia

- It is defined as the replacement of one type of cell with another type
- It is found in association with tissue damage, repair, and regeneration

○ **Examples:** Gastroesophageal reflux damages the squamous epithelium of the esophagus, replacing it with intestinal epithelium

Q4. What is hamartoma?

Ans.

Hamartomas

○ Are benign masses composed of cells indigenous to the involved site
○ For example, hamartomatous polyps seen in gastrointestinal tract

Q5. Describe the terms differentiation and anaplasia.

Ans.

Differentiation

○ Extent to which the neoplastic parenchymal cells resemble the corresponding normal parenchymal cells, both morphologically and functionally

Anaplasia: Means lack of differentiation, which is a hallmark of malignancy, and is often associated with:

○ **Pleomorphism:** Variation in size and shape of cells
○ **Abnormal nuclear morphology:** High nuclear: Cytoplasmic ratio and hyperchromasia
○ **Mitoses:** Atypical, bizarre mitotic figures
○ **Loss of polarity:** Tumor cell orientation is disturbed

Q 6. What is metastasis? Discuss in brief the different pathways of the spread of cancer.

Ans.

Metastasis

○ It is defined by the spread of the tumor to the sites that are physically discontinuous with the primary tumor
○ It is the most reliable feature which differentiates malignant from benign tumors
○ All tumors can metastasize except gliomas and basal cell carcinomas

Pathways of spread

Dissemination of cancers may occur through one of three pathways: (1) Direct seeding of body cavities or surfaces, (2) lymphatic spread, and (3) hematogenous spread

1. Seeding of body cavities and surfaces:

○ Malignant neoplasm penetrates into surrounding tissues
○ Most often involves peritoneal cavity, pleural cavity, pericardial cavity, subarachnoid and joint spaces
○ For example, mucus secreting appendiceal carcinomas fill the peritoneal cavity and is termed *pseudomyxoma peritonei*

2. Lymphatic spread:

○ Most common pathway for the initial dissemination of carcinomas
○ Sentinel lymph node: Defined as "the first node in a regional lymphatic basin that receives lymph flow from the primary tumor

○ In breast, sentinel lymph node biopsy is performed before undergoing an axillary lymph node dissection

3. Hematogenous spread

○ Seen most commonly in sarcomas

○ Liver and lungs are most frequently involved in hematogenous dissemination

○ Cancers arising in close proximity to the vertebral column embolize through the paravertebral plexus, e.g. vertebral metastases of carcinomas in the thyroid and prostate

○ Renal cell carcinoma invades the branches of the renal vein

○ Hepatocellular carcinomas often penetrate portal and hepatic veins

Points to remember

○ Breast carcinoma spreads to bone

○ Bronchogenic carcinomas involve the adrenals and the brain

○ Neuroblastomas spread to the liver and bones

Q7. Write in detail about the molecular basis of cancers.

Ans.

Molecular basis of cancer

1. Nonlethal genetic damage lies at the heart of carcinogenesis

○ Initiation of cell injury, whether induced by germline or sporadic mutation leads to genetic damage in cell, in response to which the cell genetic makeup is altered, but cell death does not occur.

2. Tumor is formed by the clonal expansion of a single precursor cell that has incurred genetic damage

○ Genetic mutations brought about in a cell are heritable and are passed on to all subset of tumor cells, hence tumors are clonal

3. Cancer causing mutations affect

○ Four classes of normal regulatory genes—growth promoting proto-oncogenes, growth-inhibiting tumor suppressor genes, genes that regulate programmed cell death (apoptosis), and genes involved in DNA repair

4. Carcinogenesis results from the accumulation of complementary mutations in a stepwise fashion over time

○ Mutations that contribute to the development of malignant phenotype are referred to as driver mutations

○ First driver mutation is the initiating mutation, in which the "initiated" cell acquire a number of additional driver mutations, which result in development of the cancer

5. In addition to tumor mutations, epigenetic aberrations (DNA methylation and histone modifications) contributes for tumor development

○ Epigenetic changes are potentially reversible by drugs that inhibit DNA- or histone-modifying factors

Q8. Write about oncogenes and their mode of activation with an example.

Ans.

Oncogenes

- Genes that promote autonomous cell growth in cancer cells
- Created by the mutations in proto-oncogenes
- Encode proteins called oncoproteins
- Oncoproteins have the ability to promote cell growth in the absence of normal growth-promoting signals
- Proto-oncogenes play a role in signaling pathways that drive proliferation
- Pro-growth proto-oncogenes encode growth factors, growth factor receptors, signal transducers, transcription factors, or cell cycle components

Mode of activation of RAS proto-oncogene and its effects

RAS Mutations

- Most common type of abnormality involving proto-oncogenes in human tumors
- Comprises HRAS, KRAS, NRAS

Normal pathway

- RAS binds guanosine nucleotides (guanosine triphosphate, GTP and guanosine diphosphate, GDP)
- Inactive RAS binds to GDP
- GDP conversion into GTP, activates RAS protein
- Activated RAS stimulates mitogen-activated protein (MAP) kinase cascade, and PI3K pathway, which signals cell proliferation
- GTP hydrolysis, converts the GTP bound, active RAS to the GDP-bound, inactive form
- GTPase activating proteins (GAPs): Increases the GTPase activity, leading to termination of signal transduction
- GAPs function as "brakes" that prevent uncontrolled RAS activity
- Mutation in neurofibromin-1, a GAP, is associated with familial neurofibromatosis type 1

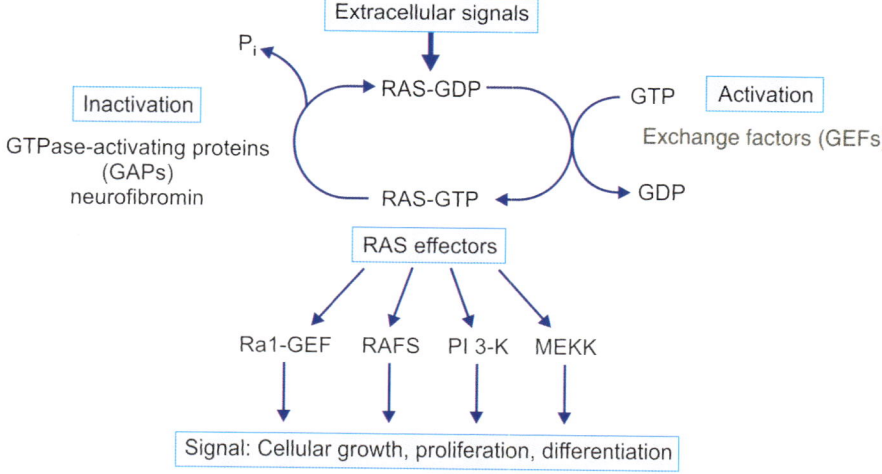

Fig. 7.1: RAS mutations

Q9. Discuss tumor suppressor genes with examples. Describe in detail about any two with their mechanisms and functions.

Ans.

Tumor suppressor genes

○ **Definition:** It is a protein or gene that is associated with suppression of any of the hallmarks of the cancer

○ Apply brakes to cell proliferation

○ Abnormalities in these genes lead to cell proliferation

Examples of tumor suppressor genes and its associations

Gene	Protein	Syndromes/Cancers
APC	Adenomatous polyposis coli protein	Familial colonic polyps and carcinomas
NF1	Neurofibromin-1	Neurofibromas, neuroblastoma, juvenile myeloid leukemia
NF2	Merlin	Acoustic schwannoma and meningioma
PTCH	Patched	Gorlin syndrome (basal cell carcinoma, medulloblastoma)
PTEN	Phosphatase and tensin homologue	Cowden syndrome, carcinomas and lymphoid tumors
SMAD 2, 4	SMAD 2, 4	Juvenile polyposis, colonic and pancreatic carcinoma
Rb.	Retinoblastoma (RB) protein	Familial retinoblastoma syndrome (retinoblastoma, osteosarcoma)
CDKN2A	p16/INK4a and p14/ARF	Melanoma, pancreatic, breast, esophageal carcinoma
VHL	von Hippel-Lindau (vHL) protein	von Hippel-Lindau syndrome (cerebellar hemangioblastoma, retinal angioma, renal cell carcinoma)
STK11	Liver kinase B1 (LKB1) or STK11	Peutz-Jeghers syndrome (GI polyps, GI cancers, pancreatic carcinoma)
CDH1	E- Cadherin	Familial gastric cancer, lobular breast carcinoma
TP53	p53 protein	Li-Fraumeni syndrome
BRCA1, BRCA2	Breast cancer-1 and breast cancer-2	Familial breast and ovarian carcinoma, carcinomas of male breast, chronic lymphocytic leukemia
MSH2, MLH1, MSH6	MSH1, MLH1, MSH6	Hereditary nonpolyposis colon carcinoma, colonic and endometrial carcinoma
WT1	Wilms' tumor-1 (WT1)	Familial Wilms' tumor
MEN1	Menin	Multiple endocrine neoplasia 1 (MEN1; pituitary, parathyroid, and pancreatic endocrine tumors)

1. *RB: Governor of proliferation*

○ Exists in an active hypophosphorylated state in quiescent cells and an inactive hyperphosphorylated state in cells passing through the G1/S cell cycle transition

○ RB phosphorylation is inhibited by cyclin-dependent kinase inhibitors (p16/INK4a)

○ Hypophosphorylated RB is in complex with E2F transcription factors, inhibits the cell to go in S phase

○ RB is phosphorylated by the cyclin D-CDK4, cyclin D-CDK6, and cyclin E-CDK2 complexes, releasing E2F, resulting in activation of S phase of cell cycle

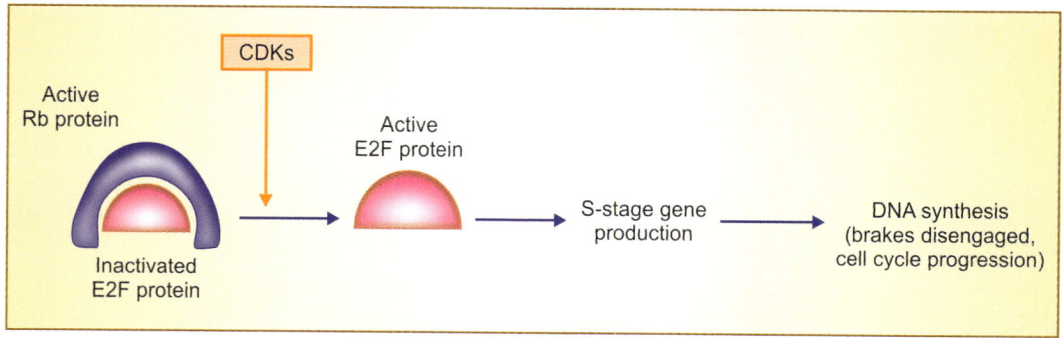

Fig. 7.2: RB protein activation

2. *TP53: Guardian of the genome*

○ Regulates cell cycle progression, DNA repair, cellular senescence, and apoptosis

○ Located on **chromosome 17p13.1**

○ Most frequently mutated gene in human cancers

○ **Li-Fraumeni syndrome:** Individuals who inherit one mutated TP53 allele, are at increased risk of developing sarcomas, breast cancer, leukemias, brain tumors, and adrenal cortical carcinomas

○ Levels of p53 are negatively regulated by MDM2

○ **HPV-E6 proteins** bind p53 and promote its degradation

p53 inhibits neoplastic transformation by:

○ Activation of temporary cell cycle arrest (quiescence), induction of permanent cell cycle arrest (senescence) or by triggering of programmed cell death (apoptosis)

p53 brings cell cycle arrest by activation of:

○ p21, GADD45 (growth arrest and DNA damage) and BAX gene

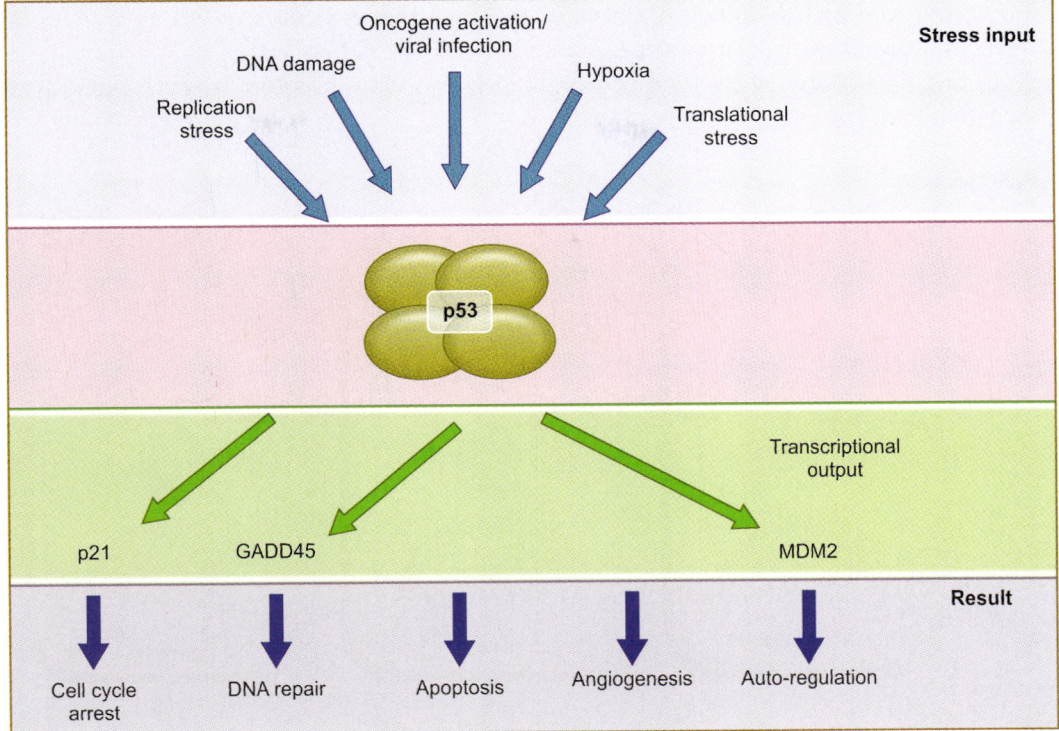

Fig. 7.3: Functions of p53

Q10. Write a short note on APC-β-catenin-WNT signaling pathway. Mention the role of E-cadherin in this pathway.

Ans.

APC: Gatekeeper of Colonic Neoplasia

- APC (5q21) gene mutation is associated with familial adenomatous polyposis
- APC and β-catenin are components of WNT signaling pathway
- In absence of WNT, APC and β-catenin in colonic epithelial cells form a macromolecular complex, resulting in destruction of β-catenin
- When colonic epithelial cells are stimulated by WNT molecules, β-catenin degradation does not occur and the later translocates to the nucleus, binds to TCF (transcription cell factor) resulting in cell cycle progression
- Also, when APC is mutated, as in colonic polyps and cancers, β-catenin translocates to the nucleus, resulting in cell cycle progression
- β-catenin, which acts as a proto-oncogene, is mutated in hepatoblastoma and hepatocellular carcinomas

E-Cadherin

- β-catenin binds to the cytoplasmic tail of E-cadherin, a cell surface protein, that maintains intercellular adhesiveness

○ Germline loss of function mutations of the E-cadherin gene, known as CDH1, is seen in familial gastric carcinoma
○ Reduced E-cadherin expression is noted in the esophagus, colon, breast, ovary, and prostate cancers

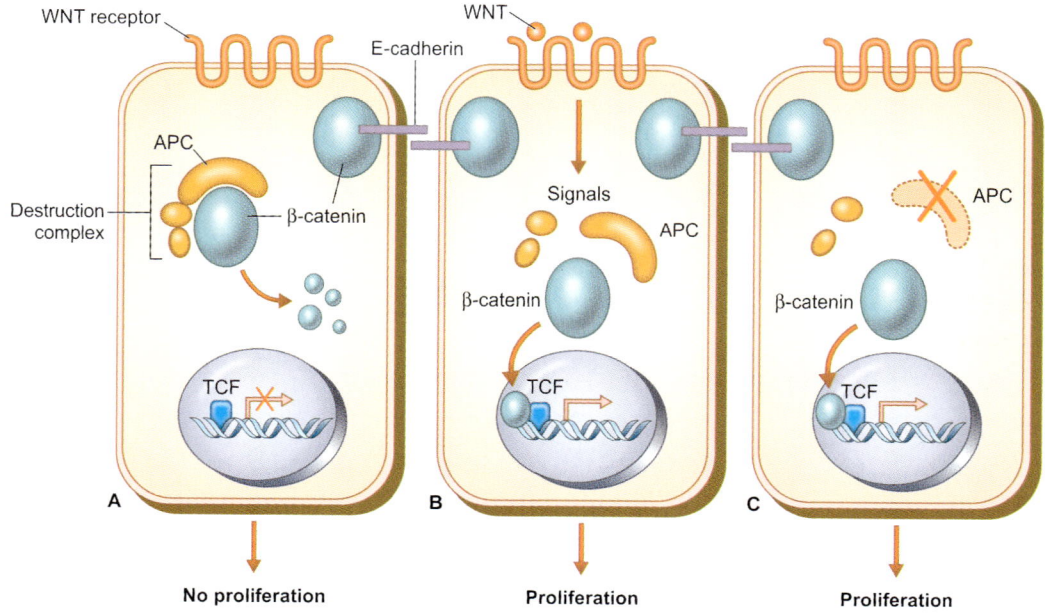

Fig. 7.4: APC β-catenin pathway

Q11. Write a short note on neurofibromatosis gene.

Ans.

Classified into two types

a. *Neurofibromatosis 1 (NF-1)*
○ Encodes neurofibromin, which is a GAP (GTPase activating protein), that acts as a brake on RAS signaling
○ Predisposes to neurofibromatosis type 1, in which patients can develop numerous benign neurofibroma and optic nerve gliomas

b. *Neurofibromatosis 2 (NF-2)*
○ Encodes neurofibromin 2 or merlin
○ Germline mutations in NF2 gene predisposes to neurofibromatosis type 2
○ Individuals with mutation in NF2 gene predisposes to benign bilateral schwannomas of the acoustic nerve, sporadic meningiomas and ependymomas

Q 12. Write a short note on Warburg effect.

Ans.

The Warburg effect
○ Cancer cells demonstrate high levels of glucose uptake

○ Cancer cells prefers aerobic glycolysis as a preferred source of energy and not oxidative phosphorylation

○ Even though oxidative phosphorylation generates 36 molecules of ATP per molecule of glucose in contrast to only 2 molecules of ATP per molecule of glucose by aerobic glycolysis

○ Aerobic glycolysis provides rapidly dividing tumor cells with metabolic intermediates that are needed for the synthesis of cellular components, whereas mitochondrial oxidative phosphorylation does not

Implication

○ "Glucose-hunger" of tumor cells is used to visualize the tumors via positron emission tomography (PET) scanning

○ In PET scanning, patients are injected with 18F-fluorodeoxyglucose, a non-metabolizable derivative of glucose that is preferentially taken up into tumor cells

Q13. Discuss in brief about autophagy.

Ans.

Autophagy

○ Severe nutrient deficiency, in which the cells arrest their growth, and cannibalize their own organelles, proteins, and membranes as carbon sources for energy production

○ Tumor cells may use autophagy to become "dormant," which allows cells to survive hard times for long periods

○ These tumor cells are resistant to therapies that kill actively dividing cells, and thus results in therapeutic failure

Q14. Write a short note on familial cancer syndromes.

Ans.

Autosomal dominant inherited cancer syndromes

Gene	Inherited predisposition
RB	Retinoblastoma
P53	Li-Fraumeni syndrome
p16INK4a	Melanoma
APC	Familial adenomatous polyposis/colon cancer
NF-1, NF-2	Neurofibromatosis 1, 2
BRCA-1, BRCA-2	Breast cancer
MEN-1, RET	Multiple endocrine neoplasia
MLH-1 and MSH-2, 6	Hereditary non-polyposis colorectal cancer
PATCH	Nevoid basal cell carcinoma syndrome

Defects in DNA repair systems like mismatch repair, nucleotide excision repair, and recombination repair—predisposes to carcinomas

Examples:

a. Hereditary nonpolyposis colon cancer syndrome:
- Occurs due to defects in DNA mismatch repair genes
- Autosomal dominant disorder, associated with familial carcinomas of the colon affecting predominantly the cecum and proximal colon
- **Microsatellite instability:** Hallmark of patients with DNA-mismatch repair genes
- Germline mutations in MSH2 and MLH1 genes are most commonly implicated

b. Xeroderma pigmentosum:
- Patients have a defect in the nucleotide excision repair pathway
- Increased risk for the development of cancers of the skin exposed to UV light

Q15. Classify chemical carcinogens and discuss in brief the steps involved in chemical carcinogenesis.

Ans.

Major chemical carcinogens

1. Direct-acting carcinogens:
   Alkylating agents
   - Anticancer drugs (cyclophosphamide, chlorambucil, nitrosoureas, and others)
   Acylating agents
   - Dimethylcarbamyl chloride

2. Procarcinogens that require metabolic activation:
   - **Polycyclic aromatic hydrocarbons:** Benzo [*a*] pyrene
   - **Aromatic amines:** Benzidine, dimethylaminoazobenzene
   - **Microbial products**: Aflatoxin B1, griseofulvin
   - **Others:** Nitrosamine and amides, vinyl chloride, nickel, chromium, insecticides, fungicides

Steps involved in chemical carcinogenesis

a. *Stage of initiation:*
   - All initiating chemical carcinogens are highly reactive electrophiles (i.e. electron-deficient atoms) that can react with nucleophilic (electron-rich) sites in the cell, i.e. DNA
   - Initiation leads to nonlethal damage to the DNA that cannot be repaired

b. *Stage of promotion/ progression during cancer development:*
   - Mutated cell passes on the DNA lesions to its daughter cells
   - Resulting in proliferation induced by promoter, with additional mutations and formation of malignant tumor

Q16. Write a short note on radiation injury.

Ans.

Radiation energy in the form of **UV rays** of sunlight or **ionizing radiation** is carcinogenic

Ultraviolet rays

- UV rays can be divided into three wavelength ranges: UVA (320–400 nm), UVB (280–320 nm), and UVC (200–280 nm)
- UVB is responsible for the induction of cutaneous cancers, e.g. **squamous cell carcinoma, basal cell carcinoma, and melanoma of the skin**
- UVB carcinogenicity is due to formation of pyrimidine dimers in DNA
- UVC, a potent mutagen, is filtered out by the ozone layer surrounding the earth

Ionizing radiation

- Electromagnetic (X-rays, λ rays) and particulate (α particles, β particles, protons, neutrons) radiations are all carcinogenic
- Predisposes to myeloid leukemias, thyroid, breast, lung and salivary glands carcinomas

Q17. Mention oncogenic viruses. Discuss in detail oncogenic DNA viruses.

Ans.

Microbial carcinogenesis

- **Oncogenic RNA viruses:** Human T-cell leukemia virus type 1
- **Oncogenic DNA Viruses:** Human papillomavirus, Epstein-Barr virus (EBV), hepatitis B virus (HBV), Merkel cell polyoma virus, and Kaposi sarcoma herpes virus (HHV-8)

1. **Human papillomavirus:**
   - **High-risk HPVs (types 16 and 18):** Implicated in squamous cell carcinomas of cervix, anogenital region, and head and neck (tonsillar mucosa)
   - **HPV-6 and HPV-11 (low-risk HPVs):** Responsible for genital warts
   - Oncogenic potential of HPV is related to products of two viral genes: **E6 and E7**

   HPV E6 protein
   - Leads to degradation of p53
   - Stimulates the expression of TERT, the catalytic subunit of telomerase

   HPV E7 protein
   - Binds to the RB protein and displaces the E2F transcription factors that are normally sequestered by RB, promoting progression through cycle
   - Inactivates the CDK inhibitors p21 and p27

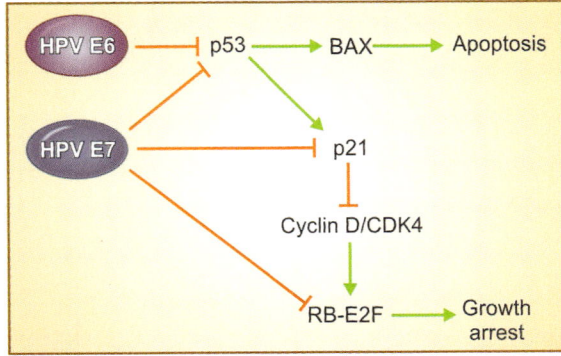

Fig. 7.5 Role of HPV in cervical carcinoma

2. **Epstein-Barr virus is implicated in pathogenesis of:**
   - ○ Burkitt lymphoma, B-cell lymphomas in immunosuppressed individuals, Hodgkin lymphoma, nasopharyngeal carcinomas, T-cell lymphoma and natural killer (NK) cell lymphoma

Points to remember:
- ○ EBV uses the complement receptor CD21 to attach to and infect B cells
- ○ EBV also possesses an oncogene, i.e. latent membrane protein-1 (LMP-1)
- ○ LMP-1 activates NF-κB and JAK/STAT signaling pathways and promotes B-cell survival and proliferation
- ○ In Burkitt lymphoma, EBV leads to acquisition of t(8;14), resulting in increased c-myc expression and resultant B-cell proliferation

Q18. Write a note on Paraneoplastic syndromes.

Ans.

Examples:

Clinical syndromes	Major forms of underlying cancer	Causal mechanism
Endocrinopathies		
Cushing syndrome	Small-cell carcinoma of lung	ACTH or ACTH-like substance
Syndrome of inappropriate antidiuretic hormone secretion	Small-cell carcinoma of lung, Intracranial neoplasms	Antidiuretic hormone/atrial natriuretic hormones
Hypercalcemia	Squamous cell carcinoma of lung, breast carcinoma, renal carcinoma, adult T-cell leukemia/lymphoma	Parathyroid hormone-related protein (PTHRP), TGF-α, TNF, IL-1
Hypoglycemia	Ovarian carcinoma, fibrosarcoma	Insulin or insulin-like substance
Polycythemia	Renal cell carcinoma, cerebellar hemangioma, hepatocellular carcinoma	Erythropoietin
Nerve and muscle syndromes		
Myasthenia	Bronchogenic carcinoma, Thymic neoplasms	Immunologic
Dermatologic Disorders		
Acanthosis nigricans	Gastric carcinoma, lung carcinoma, uterine cancer	Immunologic; secretion of epidermal growth factor
Dermatomyositis	Bronchogenic carcinoma, Breast carcinoma	Immunologic
Osseous, articular, and soft tissue changes		
Hypertrophic osteoarthropathy and clubbing of the fingers	Bronchogenic carcinoma	Unknown

Contd.

Contd.

Vascular and hematologic changes

Venous thrombosis (Trousseau phenomenon)	Pancreatic carcinoma, Bronchogenic carcinoma	Tumor products (mucins that activate clotting)
Disseminated intravascular coagulation	Acute promyelocytic leukemia, prostatic carcinoma	Tumor products that activate clotting
Nonbacterial thrombotic endocarditis	Mucin secreting adenocarcinoma	Hypercoagulability
Red cell aplasia	Thymic neoplasms	—

Q19. Write a short note on Grading and staging of tumors.

Ans.

Grade of a tumor
○ Based on the degree of differentiation of the tumor cells
○ Can be well differentiated, moderately differentiated or poorly differentiated
○ Poorly differentiated cancers show more aggressive behavior

Stage of a tumor
○ Is based on the size of the primary lesion, its extent of spread to the regional lymph nodes, and presence or absence of blood borne metastases
○ American Joint Committee on Cancer Staging (AJCC) is the major staging system currently in use
○ AJCC includes classification based on TNM system—T for primary tumor, N for regional lymph node involvement, and M for metastases

Q20. Write a short note on laboratory diagnosis of cancer.

Ans.
Lab diagnosis of cancer can be characterized into several subcategories

1. *Histological and cytological methods*
   Depends on the several sample approaches:
   a. **Excision or biopsy**:
      ○ Appropriate site of biopsy, tissue perseveration in formalin for processing and for special investigations such as cytogenetics, flow cytometry and molecular diagnostics has to be taken care of
   b. **Fine needle aspiration:**
      ○ Procedure involves aspirating cells and fluid with a small-bore needle, followed by cytological examination of the stained smear
      ○ Most commonly used for palpable lesions in breast, thyroid, and lymph nodes
   c. **Cytologic smears:**
      ○ Methods to screen carcinoma cervix patients
      ○ Also useful in endometrial carcinoma, lung carcinoma, bladder and prostatic tumors, gastric carcinomas and for identification of tumor cells in abdominal, pleural, joint, and cerebrospinal fluids

2. *Immunohistochemistry is useful in:*
- ○ Categorization of undifferentiated malignant tumors
- ○ Determination of site of origin of metastatic tumors
- ○ Detection of molecules that have prognostic or therapeutic significance, e.g. estrogen receptor and progesterone receptor positivity in breast cancers

3. *Flow cytometry:* useful in B- and T-cell lymphomas and leukemias

4. *Molecular and cytogenetic diagnostics*:
- ○ Diagnosis of malignant neoplasms
- ○ Prognosis of malignant neoplasms
- ○ Detection of minimal residual disease
- ○ Diagnosis of hereditary predisposition to cancer

Q21. Enumerate major tumor markers with examples.

Ans.

Tumor markers	Tumor types
Hormones	
Human chorionic gonadotropin	Trophoblastic tumors, nonseminomatous testicular tumors
Calcitonin	Medullary carcinoma of thyroid
Catecholamine	Pheochromocytoma
Oncofetal antigens	
α-Fetoprotein	Liver cell cancer, nonseminomatous germ cell tumors of testis
Carcinoembryonic antigen (CEA)	Carcinomas of the colon, pancreas, lung, stomach, and heart
Isoenzymes	
Prostatic acid phosphatase	Prostate cancer
Neuron-specific enolase	Small-cell cancer of lung, neuroblastoma
Specific proteins	
Immunoglobulins	Multiple myeloma and other gammopathies
Prostate-specific antigen	Prostate cancer
Mucins and other glycoproteins	
CA-125	Ovarian cancer
CA-19-9	Colon cancer, pancreatic cancer
CA-15-3	Breast cancer
Cell-free DNA markers	
TP53, APC, RAS mutants in stool and serum	Colon cancer
TP53, RAS mutants in stool and serum	Pancreatic cancer
TP53, RAS mutants in sputum and serum	Lung cancer
TP53 mutants in urine	Bladder cancer

8

Infectious Diseases

Q1. What are Warthin-Finkeldey giant cells?

Ans.

Warthin-Finkeldey cells

○ Pathognomonic of measles
○ Multinucleate giant cells, comprising of eosinophilic intra-nuclear and cytoplasmic inclusion bodies
○ Found in the lung and sputum

Note: Koplik spots: Ulcerated mucosal lesions in the oral cavity near the opening of the Stensen ducts, seen in measles

Q2. Write a note on tertiary syphilis.

Ans.

Causative organism: Treponema pallidum

Three stages:

1. **Primary syphilis**
   ○ Characterized by single firm, non-tender, raised, red lesion (chancre)
   ○ Sites: Penis, cervix, vaginal wall, or anus
   ○ Chancre can heal with or without therapy

2. **Secondary syphilis**
   ○ Seen in untreated primary syphilis patients
   ○ Presents as painless, superficial lesions on palms or soles of the feet, oral cavity, vagina
   ○ Lymphadenopathy, condyloma latum are associated findings
   ○ Asymptomatic neurosyphilis can also be seen in a few patients

3. **Tertiary syphilis**
   ○ **Three manifestations:** Cardiovascular syphilis, neurosyphilis, benign tertiary syphilis
   ○ **Cardiovascular syphilis:** Presents as aneurysms and aortic regurgitation

○ **Neurosyphilis:** Symptomatic or asymptomatic, asymptomatic neurosyphilis is diagnosed by CSF pleocytosis (increased cell count), elevated protein levels, decreased glucose levels
○ **Benign tertiary syphilis:** Characterized by gumma formation in liver (hepar lobatum), bone, skin and mucous membranes. Gummas are nodular lesions, due to development of delayed hypersensitivity to the bacteria

Note
○ Congenital syphilis include a **triad of interstitial keratitis, Hutchinson teeth, and eighth nerve deafness**

Q3. Write a note on viral hemorrhagic fevers.

Ans.
○ It is a severe life-threatening multisystem syndrome, characterized by vascular dysregulation and damage, leading to shock
○ Symptoms range from fever, headache, myalgia, rash, neutropenia, thrombocytopenia to severe life-threatening disease
○ Causative agent: RNA viruses: Arenaviridae, Filoviridae, Bunyaviridae, and Flaviviridae
○ Caused by direct infection and damage to endothelial cells

Q4. Write a note on Rhinosporidiosis.

Ans.
Rhinosporidiosis
○ Causative agent: *Rhinosporidium seeberi*
○ Characterized by hyperplastic polypoid lesions of the nasal cavity

Microscopy
○ Large globular cysts are present surrounded by a heavy inflammatory reaction
○ Each of these cysts represents a thick-walled sporangium containing numerous spores

9

Environment and Nutritional Diseases

Q1. Write a note on vitamin A deficiency

Ans.

Causes of vitamin A deficiency
In children: Infections
In adults: Celiac disease, Crohn disease, Colitis

Manifestations
○ Night blindness, epithelial metaplasia and keratinization
○ Xerophthalmia (dry eye)
○ **Bitot spots:** Opaque plaques on corneal surface, which progresses to erosion and resulting in keratomalacia and blindness
○ **Immune deficiency:** Responsible for infections (measles, pneumonia, and diarrhea)

Q2. Write a note on vitamin C deficiency.

Ans.

Risk factors
○ Seen in chronic alcoholics, individuals with poor diets, older individuals, patients undergoing peritoneal dialysis and hemodialysis

Vitamin C deficiency (scurvy)
Results in impaired collagen formation, which leads to:
a. Bleeding tendency
b. Inadequate synthesis of osteoid
c. Impaired wound healing

Q3. Write a note on trace elements and their deficiency states.

Ans.

Element	Clinical features
Zinc	Acrodermatitis enteropathica, anorexia and diarrhea, growth retardation, impaired wound healing, impaired night vision, infertility

Contd.

Contd.

Iron	Microcytic hypochromic anemia
Iodine	Goiter and hypothyroidism
Copper	Muscle weakness, neurologic defects, abnormal collagen cross-linking
Fluoride	Dental caries
Selenium	Myopathy, cardiomyopathy (Keshan disease)

Q4. Write a note on kwashiorkor.

Ans.

Kwashiorkor

- Most common form of protein energy malnutrition (PEM)
- Most commonly seen in African nations
- Generalized or dependent edema: Due to marked protein loss
- Skin lesions: Alternating zones of hyperpigmentation, areas of desquamation, and hypopigmentation, giving a **"flaky paint" appearance**
- Hair changes: Loss of color or alternating bands of pale and darker hair
- Fatty liver
- Defects in immunity and secondary infections

Morphology

- **Small bowel** shows mucosal atrophy with loss of villi
- **Bone marrow:** Appears hypocellular
- **Peripheral blood smear:** Anemia can be microcytic, normocytic, or macrocytic or anemia of chronic disease
- **Brain:** Cerebral atrophy
- Thymic and lymphoid atrophy
- Parasitic and worm infestations

Q5. Write a note on rickets.

Ans.

Rickets

- Normal reference range for circulating 25-hydroxycholecalciferol 25-(OH)-D is 20 to 100 ng/ml
- Concentrations of less than 20 ng/ml constitute vitamin D deficiency, termed rickets in growing children and osteomalacia in adults

Morphology of bones in rickets

- Failure of the cartilage cells to mature, resulting in the deposition of immature cartilage (unmineralized bone deposition), which predisposes to repeated fractures
- Frontal bossing of the head

○ Rachitic rosary: Deformation of the chest wall (pigeon breast deformity)
○ Lumbar lordosis and bowing of the legs

Note
○ On microscopy, unmineralized osteoid stains pink in hematoxylin and eosin preparations, whereas normally mineralized trabeculae are more basophilic

Q6. Write a note on obesity.

Ans.

Obesity
○ Predisposes to increased incidence of type 2 diabetes, dyslipidemias, cardiovascular disease, hypertension, and cancer

Important points to remember
○ Individuals with BMI more than 30 kg/m² are classified as obese
○ Central obesity is associated with increased incidence of number of diseases
○ Appetite and satiety are under control of leptin, adiponetion and gut hormones
○ Gut hormones include ghrelin, pancreatic polypeptide, insulin, and amylin
○ **Ghrelin**—produced in stomach and hypothalamus—**increases food intake**
○ **Amylin**—**reduces food intake** and weight gain

10

Diseases of Infancy and Childhood

Q1. Write a short note on neonatal respiratory distress syndrome.

Ans.

Respiratory distress syndrome (RDS)/hyaline membrane disease
- Seen in **preterm infants**
- Associated with male gender
- Risk factors: Maternal diabetes, cesarean section
- Predisposing factor—lung immaturity
- Incidence of RDS is inversely proportional to the gestational age
- Fundamental defect in RDS is deficiency of pulmonary surfactant
- Surfactant synthesis is increased by cortisol, insulin, prolactin, thyroxine, TGF-β and is suppressed by insulin
- Labor increases surfactant synthesis
- Microscopically, **eosinophilic hyaline membranes** line the **respiratory bronchioles**, alveolar ducts, and alveoli

Complications due to treatment of RDS
- High concentration and prolonged oxygen administration leads to retrolental fibroplasia (also called retinopathy of prematurity) and bronchopulmonary dysplasia

Q2. Write a note on hemolytic disease of newborn.

Ans.

Hemolytic disease of newborn (immune hydrops)
- Caused by blood group antigen incompatibility between mother and fetus
- Rh and ABO blood groups antigens can induce clinically significant immunologic reactions

Etiology and Pathogenesis
- Occurs when fetal red cells reach maternal circulation
- Results in antibody response
- Among the Rh antigens, **D antigen** is a major cause of Rh incompatibility

- Initial exposure to Rh antigen, result in **IgM antibodies** formation
- **Rh disease** is uncommon after **first pregnancy**
- However, during **subsequent pregnancy** (due to **IgG antibody** response), risk of **immune hydrops** is increased

How to protect?

- **Anti-D antibodies (RhIg)** usage has reduced the incidence of maternal Rh iso-immunization
- Administration of RhIg to the mother is done at 28 weeks of pregnancy and within 72 hours of delivery
- RhIg is also administered following abortions
- Immunization to Rh negative mothers decreases the risk for hemolytic disease in Rh-positive neonates in subsequent pregnancies

Q3. Write a short note on ABO incompatibility.

Ans.

ABO incompatibility

- Seen in 20% to 25% of pregnancies
- **Anti-A** and **anti-B antibodies** produced are of IgM type, which do not cross the placenta
- Disease is milder than Rh incompatibility
- There is no effective protection against ABO reactions

Disease is not as severe as Rh incompatibility because

- Neonatal red cells express blood group antigens A and B poorly
- Cells, other than red cells, express A and B antigens, which absorbs some of the transferred antibody

Whom does it affect and why?

- ABO hemolytic disease affects infants with group A or B, who are born to group O mothers
- For some unknown reasons, group O women possess IgG antibodies directed against group A or B antigens, even without prior sensitization, resulting in affected first child

Q4. Write a note on erythroblastosis fetalis.

Ans.

Erythroblastosis fetalis

- In immune hydrops, fetus will be severely anemic
- Liver and spleen will be enlarged, due to cardiac failure, secondary to anemia
- In bone marrow, there occurs compensatory hyperplasia of the erythroid precursors
- Extramedullary hematopoiesis is present in liver, spleen, and lymph nodes
- Increased hematopoietic activity results in increased numbers of immature red cells, including reticulocytes, normoblasts, and erythroblasts **(erythroblastosis fetalis)**

Q5. Write a note on etiopathogenesis of cystic fibrosis.

Ans.

Cystic fibrosis

- Disorder of ion transport in epithelial cells
- Affects fluid secretion in exocrine glands and epithelial lining of the respiratory, gastrointestinal, and reproductive tracts
- Results from abnormal function of epithelial chloride channel protein encoded by **cystic fibrosis trans-membrane conductance regulator (CFTR) gene**
- CFTR gene is located on chromosome 7q31.2
- Pulmonary manifestations are associated with mutation of mannose-binding lectin 2 (MBL2) and transforming growth factor β1 (TGFB1)

Q6. Enumerate the tumors affecting children.

Ans.

Tumors commonly encountered in childhood

- Leukemia, teratomas, Ewing sarcoma, rhabdomyosarcomas, hepatoblastoma, Wilms' tumor, osteogenic sarcoma, neuroblastoma, retinoblastoma

Q7. Discuss neuroblastoma in relation to its clinical features, morphology and its prognostic factors.

Ans.

Neuroblastomas

- Most common extra-cranial solid tumor of childhood
- Associated with germline mutations in **anaplastic lymphoma kinase (ALK)** gene
- **Sites:** Adrenal gland (40%), along the sympathetic chain, i.e. paravertebral region of the abdomen (25%) and posterior mediastinum
- Tumors can show spontaneous regression

Gross

- Range in size from **minute nodules to large masses**

Microscopy

- Tumor cells, arranged in solid sheets, have scant cytoplasm with dark nuclei
- Background demonstrates faintly eosinophilic fibrillary material (neuropil)
- **Homer Wright pseudo rosettes**—tumor cells are concentrically arranged about a central space filled with neuropil
- **Ganglioneuroblastoma:** Composed of ganglion cells (cells with abundant cytoplasm, large vesicular nuclei, and prominent nucleolus) admixed with primitive neuroblasts
- **Ganglioneuromas:** Better differentiated lesions, with mature ganglion cells and a few neuroblasts
- Maturation of neuroblasts into ganglion cells is accompanied by the appearance of Schwann cells
- Schwannian stroma indicates a favorable outcome

Prognostic factors in neuroblastomas

Variable	Favorable	Unfavorable
Age	<18 months	>18 months
Evidence of schwannian stroma and gangliocytic differentiation	Present	Absent
DNA ploidy	Hyper diploid or near triploid	Near diploid
N-MYC	Not amplified	Amplified
Chromosome 17q gain	Absent	Present
Chromosome 1p loss	Absent	Present
Chromosome 11q loss	Absent	Present
TRKA expression	Present	Absent
TRKB expression	Absent	Present
Telomerase expression	Low or absent	Highly expressed

N-MYC amplification—most important prognostic marker

Q8. Write a note on genetics and morphology of Wilms' tumor.

Ans.

Pathogenesis and genetics

Risk is increased in any of the four groups of congenital malformations

1. **WAGR syndrome**
   - Characterized by Wilms' tumor, aniridia, genital anomalies, and mental retardation
   - Individuals carry germline deletions of 11p13
   - Patients with aniridia shows PAX6 gene mutations

2. **Denys-Drash syndrome**
   - Characterized by male pseudohermaphroditism, and diffuse mesangial sclerosis
   - Patients show germline abnormalities in WT1
   - Increased risk for developing germ cell tumors (gonadoblastoma)

3. **Beckwith-Wiedemann syndrome**
   - Characterized by enlargement of body organs (organomegaly), macroglossia, hemihypertrophy, omphalocele, and abnormal large cells in the adrenal cortex (adrenal cytomegaly)
   - Chromosomal region implicated—localized to band 11p15.5 ("WT2")
   - Increased risk for developing hepatoblastoma, pancreatoblastoma, adrenocortical tumors, and rhabdomyosarcoma

Morphology of Wilms' tumor

Gross

- Present as large, solitary, well-circumscribed mass
- 10% are bilateral or multicentric at the time of diagnosis

Cut section

○ Tumor is soft, homogeneous, and tan to gray with occasional foci of hemorrhage, cyst formation, and necrosis

Microscopy

○ Classic tri-phasic combination of blastemal, stromal, and epithelial cell types are seen
○ Blastemal component: Sheets of small blue cells
○ Epithelial differentiation: In the form of abortive tubules or glomeruli
○ Stromal cells: Fibrocystic or myxoid in nature

11

Blood Vessels and Cardiovascular System

Q1. Write a short note on heart failure cells and conditions associated with it.

Ans.

In order to learn this entity, one should be thorough with left heart failure and its predisposing conditions.

Left heart failure
Causes: Ischemic heart disease, hypertension, aortic and mitral valvular diseases, primary myocardial diseases

Effects of left-sided heart failure
- Blood backing up in the pulmonary circulation
- Stasis of blood in left-sided chambers
- Inadequate perfusion of downstream tissues leading to organ dysfunction

Morphology
Heart
- Left ventricle is hypertrophied and dilated
- Impaired left ventricle function, which predisposes to atrial fibrillation

Lungs
- Peri-vascular and interstitial edema, responsible for the characteristic Kerley B and C lines on chest X-ray
- Accumulation of edema fluid in alveolar spaces and widening of the alveolar septae
- Alveolar macrophages within alveolar spaces engulf hemosiderin and results in formation of hemosiderin-laden macrophages (heart failure cells)
- **Heart failure cells** are stained by Perl's/Prussian blue stain

Q2. Write a short note on cor pulmonale.

Ans.
Pulmonary (right-sided) hypertensive heart disease (cor pulmonale)
- Occurs due to the right ventricular pressure overload

Chronic cor pulmonale
- **Causes:** Chronic parenchymal lung diseases such as emphysema, and primary pulmonary hypertension
- Characterized by right ventricular hypertrophy, dilation, and right-sided failure
- Right ventricular wall thickens, up to 1.0 cm or more

Acute cor pulmonale
- Can follow massive pulmonary embolism
- Characterized by marked dilation of right ventricle without hypertrophy
- **Cross-section:** Normal crescent shape of right ventricle is transformed to a dilated ovoid shape

Q3. Write a short note on tetralogy of Fallot.

Ans.

Tetralogy of Fallot (TOF)
4 cardinal features of TOF
- Ventricular septal defect
- Obstruction of the right ventricular outflow tract (sub-pulmonary stenosis)
- An aorta that overrides the ventricular septal defect (VSD)
- Right ventricular hypertrophy

Morphology
- Boot-shaped heart—due to marked right ventricular hypertrophy
- Large VSD, with the aortic valve at the superior border
- Right ventricular outflow tract obstruction—due to sub-pulmonic stenosis or pulmonary valvular stenosis
- Right aortic arch is present in 25% of cases

Clinical features
- **Classic TOF**—severe right ventricular outflow tract obstruction, leads to right-to-left shunting, producing cyanosis
- **Pink tetralogy**—left to right shunt, mild sub-pulmonary stenosis, does not produce cyanosis

Q4. Write a short note on coarctation of aorta.

Ans.

Coarctation of aorta
- Male:Female :: 2:1
- Two forms: Infantile form and adult form

a. *Coarctation of the aorta with PDA (infantile form)*
- Produces signs and symptoms immediately after birth
- There occurs tubular hypoplasia of the aortic arch, which occurs proximal to patent ductus arteriosus
- Presents as cyanosis localized to the lower half of the body

b. *Coarctation of the aorta without a PDA (adult form)*
○ Asymptomatic in childhood, presents in adult life
○ Presents as a ridge like infolding of the aorta just opposite the closed ductus arteriosus (ligamentum arteriosum)
○ Can cause hypertension in upper extremities and hypotension in lower extremities

X-ray finding: Development of collateral circulation between pre-coarctation and post-coarctation arteries (through enlarged inter-coastal and internal mammary arteries), thus producing notching of the undersurfaces of ribs.

Q5. Define atherosclerosis. Discuss the morphology of atheroma, risk factors and complications associated with atherosclerosis.

Ans.
Definition: Atherosclerosis is characterized by intimal lesions called atheromas, or atheromatous or fibrofatty plaques, which protrude into and obstruct vascular lumens and weaken the underlying media.

Risk factors:
○ **Non-modifiable risk factors:** Age: 40–60 years, Sex: M > F, genetic predisposition
○ **Modifiable risk factors:** Hyperlipidemia, hypertension, cigarette smoking, diabetes mellitus
○ **Inflammation:** Increased CRP expression is a risk factor for MI, stroke, peripheral arterial disease. CRP is produced in liver and is stimulated by increased IL-6 levels
○ **Hyperhomocystinemia** (>100 μmol/L), sedentary lifestyle, obesity, type A personality

Morphology of an Atheroma
a. Fibrous cap: Composed of smooth muscle cells (SMCs), connective tissue, a few leucocytes
b. Shoulder (cellular area beneath and to the side of the cap): Composed of smooth muscle cells, macrophages, lymphocytes
c. Necrotic zone: Disorganized mass of lipid material, cholesterol clefts, cellular debris, lipid laden foam cells, fibrin, thrombi
d. Neovascularisation at periphery

Atherosclerotic plaques can undergo following pathological changes:
a. Rupture, ulceration, or erosion in a plaque exposes highly thrombogenic substances and leads to thrombosis which may occlude the vessel lumen
b. Hemorrhage into a plaque: Occurs due to the rupture of the overlying fibrous cap, or thin-walled vessels in the areas of neovascularization
c. Embolism: Plaque rupture can produce thromboembolism
d. Aneurysm formation: Atherosclerosis-induced pressure atrophy of the underlying media

Consequences of atherosclerotic disease:
○ Myocardial infarction, cerebral infarction, aortic aneurysms, and peripheral vascular disease (gangrene of the legs)

Q6. Write a short note on aneurysms.

Ans.

Aneurysm

Definition: Localized abnormal dilation of the blood vessel or heart

Types

a. True aneurysm:
- Aneurysm involving thinned out intact arterial wall or thinned ventricular wall of the heart
- **Examples:** Atherosclerotic, syphilitic, congenital vascular aneurysms or the ventricular aneurysms that follow transmural myocardial infarctions

b. False aneurysm (pseudoaneurysm):
- Defect in the vascular wall leading to an extravascular hematoma, which communicates within the intravascular space
- **Example:** Ventricular rupture after myocardial infarction, contained by a pericardial adhesion

Classification of aneurysms
- **Saccular aneurysms:** Spherical outpouching involving only a portion of the vessel wall; can vary from 5 to 20 cm in diameter and often contain thrombus
- **Fusiform aneurysms:** Diffuse, circumferential dilation of a long vascular segment; can vary up to 20 cm in diameter

Causes
- Two most important causes of aortic aneurysms are atherosclerosis and hypertension
- **Atherosclerosis** is a risk factor for abdominal aortic aneurysms
- **Hypertension** is the most common etiology associated with ascending aortic aneurysms
- **Other causes:** Trauma, vasculitis, fibromuscular dysplasia, infections (mycotic aneurysms)

Q7. A 50-year-old man collapses suddenly while climbing the stairs with severe chest pain and profuse sweating.

a. What is your clinical diagnosis?

b. Enlist the biochemical tests and their role in diagnosis of this disease.

c. Discuss the evolution of morphologic changes in myocardial infarction.

Ans.

a. Myocardial infarction

b. Lab findings in myocardial ischemia
- Measuring blood levels of proteins that leak out of irreversibly damaged myocytes
- Most useful of these molecules are cardiac specific troponins T and I (cTnT and cTnI), and CK-MB
- Most sensitive and specific biomarkers of myocardial damage are cardiac-specific proteins, particularly cTnT and cTnI
- Troponins I and T are not normally detectable in the circulation

1. *Troponin T:*
   - ○ Begins to rise within 3–12 hours of the onset of MI, peaks at 12–48 hours and return back to normal within 5–14 days

2. *Troponin I:*
   - ○ Begins to rise within 3–12 hours of the onset of MI, peaks at 24 hours and return back to normal within 5–10 days

3. *Creatinine kinase MB:*
   - ○ Begins to rise within 3–12 hours of the onset of MI, peaks at 24 hours, and returns to normal within 48 to 72 hours

Evolution of morphological changes in myocardial infarction:

Reversible injury		
Time	Gross features	Microscopy
0–½ hour	None	None
Irreversible injury		
½–4 hours	None	Waviness of fibers
4–12 hours	Dark mottling (occasional)	Coagulation necrosis; edema; hemorrhage
12–24 hours	Dark mottling	Ongoing coagulation necrosis, early infiltration by neutrophils
1–3 days	Mottling with yellow-tan infarct at the center	Coagulation necrosis, brisk interstitial infiltrate of neutrophils
3–7 days	Hyperemic border; central yellow-tan softening	Disintegration of dead myofibers, early phagocytosis of dead cells by macrophages at infarct border
7–10 days	Maximally yellow-tan and soft, with depressed red-tan margins	Well-developed phagocytosis of dead cells; early granulation tissue at margins
10–14 days	Red-gray depressed infarct borders	Well-established granulation tissue with collagen deposition
2–8 weeks	Gray-white scar	Increased collagen deposition, with decreased cellularity
>2 months	Scarring complete	Dense collagenous scar

Q8. Enumerate the complications following myocardial infarction.

Ans.

Complications following acute myocardial infarction–
- ○ **Contractile dysfunction**—leads to left ventricular failure, cardiogenic shock
- ○ **Arrhythmias**—sinus bradycardia, heart block (asystole), tachycardia, ventricular premature contractions or ventricular tachycardia and ventricular fibrillation
- ○ **Myocardial rupture**—**anterolateral ventricular free wall** (most common), **ventricular septum** (less common), and **papillary muscle** (least common)

○ **Pericarditis** – fibrinohemorrhagic pericarditis **(Dressler syndrome)**
○ Mural thrombus and thromboembolism

Q9. Discuss etio-pathogenesis, pathologic lesions, laboratory diagnosis, clinical features and complications of rheumatic heart disease (RHD).

Ans.

Rheumatic fever (RF)

○ Multisystem inflammatory disorder occurring within a few weeks after an episode of group A streptococcal pharyngitis
○ Involves most commonly mitral valve
○ RHD is the only cause of mitral stenosis

Pathogenesis

○ Results from host immune responses to group A streptococcal antigens
○ Antibodies and CD4+ T cells against these antigens can cross-react with cardiac self-antigens
○ Binding of the antibody can activate complement, macrophages and neutrophils
○ Also seen is the cytokine mediated macrophage activation (within Aschoff body)

Morphology

In acute RF, focal inflammatory lesions are seen

○ **Aschoff bodies:** These consist of T-lymphocytes, plasma cells and plump activated macrophages called **Anitschkow cells** (pathognomonic for RF)
○ Macrophages have abundant cytoplasm and central round-to-ovoid nuclei in which the chromatin condenses into a central, slender, wavy ribbon ("caterpillar cells")
○ **Pancarditis:** Inflammation and Aschoff bodies can be seen in endocardium, pericardium and myocardium
○ **Endocardium:** 1–2 mm vegetations along the lines of closure of valve called verrucae
○ **MacCallum plaques:** Irregular thickenings seen in subendocardial regions in left atrium

Clinical features

Major manifestations

○ Migratory polyarthritis of the large joints
○ Pancarditis
○ Subcutaneous nodules
○ Erythema marginatum of the skin
○ Sydenham chorea (involuntary rapid, purposeless movements)

Minor manifestations:

○ Fever, arthralgia, or elevated blood levels of acute phase reactants

Diagnosis requires 2 major manifestations or one major and two minor manifestations, with evidence of preceding group A streptococcal infection

Complications

o Mitral valve in chronic RHD: Leaflet thickening, commissural fusion, thickening and fusion of the chordae tendineae
o "Fish mouth" or "buttonhole" stenosis: Of mitral valve is a characteristic feature of RHD.

Q10. Discuss etio-pathogenesis and morphology of heart lesions in infective endocarditis.

Ans.

Infective endocarditis

o Characterized by microbial infection of the heart valves or the mural endocardium
o Results in the formation of vegetations composed of thrombotic debris and organisms, associated with destruction of the underlying cardiac tissues
o Most common etiology—bacterial

Etiology and pathogenesis

o **Predisposing factors:** Rheumatic heart disease (in past), mitral valve prolapse, calcific valvular stenosis, bicuspid aortic valve
o *Staphylococcus aureus* can infect healthy or deformed valves
o *Staphylococcus aureus* is the major offender among intravenous drug abusers
o *Streptococcus viridans* infects deformed valve or previously damaged valves
o *Staphylococcus epidermidis*—predisposes to prosthetic valve endocarditis
o **HACEK** group (Haemophilus, Actinobacillus, Cardiobacterium, Eikenella, and Kingella) and enterococi also leads to IE

Morphology

o Vegetations on heart valves are the classic hallmark of IE
o Vegetations are friable, bulky, potentially destructive lesions containing fibrin, inflammatory cells, and bacteria
o Most common sites of infection: Aortic and mitral valves
o Ring abscess: Vegetations can be single or multiple and can erode into the underlying myocardium and produce an abscess
o Vegetations are prone to embolization
o Septic infarcts or mycotic aneurysms: Abscesses develop at the sites, where the emboli lodge

Q11. Write a short note on Libman-Sacks endocarditis.

Ans.

Libman-Sacks disease

o Seen rarely in SLE
o Characterized by small, sterile vegetations on mitral and tricuspid valves
o Vegetations are small (1 to 4 mm in diameter), single or multiple, sterile with a warty (verrucous) appearance

○ Vegetations are located on the undersurfaces of the atrioventricular valves, on the valvular endocardium, on the chords or on mural endocardium of atria or ventricles

○ **Libman-Sacks endocarditis:** When the vegetations are associated with fibrinoid necrosis of the valve substance (valvulitis)

Q12. Write a note on dilated cardiomyopathy, with a mention about its morphology and complications.

Ans.

Dilated cardiomyopathy (DCM)

○ Characterized by progressive cardiac dilation and systolic dysfunction, with concomitant hypertrophy

Pathogenesis

a. *Genetic influences*

○ Mutations in TTN, a gene that encodes titin accounts for 20% of all cases of DCM

○ Most common inheritance pattern: Autosomal dominant (AD)

b. *Myocarditis*

○ Coxsackie B virus

c. *Alcohol abuse:* *Alcohol and its metabolite, acetaldehyde is toxic to myocardium*

d. *Drugs:* *Doxorubicin, cobalt, tyrosine kinase inhibitors*

e. *Childbirth*

○ **Peripartum cardiomyopathy** can occur late in pregnancy

○ Because of ischemic injury to the myocardium

f. *Iron overload*

g. *Supraphysiologic stress:* Persistent tachycardia, hyperthyroidism, in the fetuses of insulin dependent diabetic mothers

Morphology

○ Heart is enlarged, heavy (often weighing two to three times normal), and flabby, due to dilation of all chambers

○ Mural thrombi are common

○ Most of the muscle cells are hypertrophied with enlarged nuclei

○ Interstitial and endocardial fibrosis is present

Q13. Enumerate the causes of myocarditis. Discuss its morphological features.

Ans.

Major causes of myocarditis

1. Infections

○ Viruses (e.g. coxsackievirus, influenza, HIV, cytomegalovirus)

○ Chlamydiae (e.g. *Chlamydia psittaci*)

○ Rickettsiae (e.g. *Rickettsia typhi*, typhus fever)

○ Bacteria (e.g. *Corynebacterium diphtheriae, Neisseria meningococcus*, Borrelia, Lyme disease)

○ Fungi (e.g. Candida)

○ Protozoa (e.g. *Trypanosoma cruzi* [Chagas disease], toxoplasmosis)

○ Helminths (e.g. trichinosis)

2. Immune-mediated reactions

○ Postviral

○ Poststreptococcal (rheumatic fever)

○ Systemic lupus erythematosus

○ Drug hypersensitivity (e.g. methyldopa, sulfonamides)

○ Transplant rejection

3. Unknown

○ Sarcoidosis

○ Giant cell myocarditis

Morphology

○ **Active myocarditis:** Diffuse, mononuclear cell (lymphocyte) infiltrate is seen

○ **Hypersensitivity myocarditis:** Interstitial infiltrates, composed of lymphocytes, macrophages, and eosinophils

○ **Giant cell myocarditis:** Characterized by a widespread inflammatory infiltrate containing multinucleate giant cells (fused macrophages) interspersed with lymphocytes, eosinophils, plasma cells, and macrophages with focal to extensive necrosis

○ **Myocarditis in Chagas disease:** Myofibers are distended with trypanosomes

Q14. Write a short note on cardiac myxoma.

Ans.

Myxomas

○ Most common primary tumor of the adult heart

○ Arises from primitive multipotent mesenchymal cells

○ 90% arise in the atria, most commonly in left atria

Morphology

○ Can be single or multiple

○ **Site:** Fossa ovalis in the atrial septum

○ **Size:** Varies from <1 cm to ≥10 cm, can be sessile or pedunculated lesions

○ **Gross:** Globular hard masses with hemorrhagic to soft, translucent, papillary, or villous lesions

○ **Microscopy:** Myxomas are composed of stellate or globular myxoma cells, which are embedded in an abundant mucopolysaccharide ground substance. Peculiar vessel-like or gland-like structures are characteristic

○ Hemorrhage and mononuclear inflammatory cell infiltrate are present

Q15. Classify vasculitis and write a short note on Takayasu's arteritis.

Ans.

1. Large vessel vasculitis
- Giant cell arteritis
- Takayasu arteritis

2. Medium vessel vasculitis
- Polyarteritis nodosa
- Kawasaki disease

3. Small vessel vasculitis
- **a. ANCA associated vasculitis:** Microscopic polyangiitis, Wegener granulomatosis, Churg-Strauss syndrome
- **b. Immune complex mediated vasculitis:** SLE, Henoch-Schönlein purpura, cryoglobuin vasculitis, Goodpasture's disease

Takayasu arteritis
- Age group: Less than 50 years
- Granulomatous vasculitis of medium and larger arteries
- Characterized by ocular disturbances and marked weakening of the pulses in the upper extremities (pulse less disease)

Morphology
- Involves aortic arch, pulmonary artery, coronary and renal arteries
- Microscopically, tunica media is destroyed by mononuclear inflammatory cells and giant cells

Clinical features
- Reduced blood pressure and weak pulses in carotids and upper extremities, ocular disturbances, total blindness, neurologic deficits
- Claudication of the legs, pulmonary hypertension

Q16. Write a short note on microscopic polyangiitis.

Ans.

Microscopic polyangiitis
- Also called hypersensitivity vasculitis or leukocytoclastic vasculitis
- Necrotizing vasculitis affecting the capillaries, small arterioles and venules
- All lesions tend to be of same age in the patient
- Necrotizing glomerulonephritis and pulmonary capillaritis are common

Associations
- Henoch-Schönlein purpura, essential mixed cryoglobulinemia, and vasculitis associated with connective tissue disorders

Pathogenesis
- Associated with MPO-ANCA

Morphology

- **Leukocytoclastic vasculitis:** Fragmentation of neutrophils in and around blood vessel walls
- Focal fibrinoid necrosis or transmural inflammation can be seen

Clinical features

- Hemoptysis, hematuria and proteinuria, bowel pain or bleeding, palpable cutaneous purpura

Q17. Write a short note on Wegener granulomatosis.

Ans.

Granulomatosis with polyangiitis (Wegener granulomatosis)

Triad of:

- Necrotizing granuloma of the upper respiratory tract (ear, nose, sinuses, throat) or the lower respiratory tract (lung) or both
- Necrotizing or granulomatous vasculitis affecting small to medium-sized vessels, in the lungs and upper airways (most common)
- Crescentic glomerulonephritis

Pathogenesis

- PR3-ANCAs are present in 95% of cases, useful marker of disease activity

Morphology

a. **Lung lesion:** Large nodular centrally cavitating lesions

b. **Renal lesions:**
  - Focal and segmental necrotizing glomerulonephritis
  - Parietal cell proliferation resulting in formation of crescents **(crescentic glomerulonephritis)**

c. **Arterial lesions:** Vasculitis of small artery with adjacent granulomatous inflammation including epithelioid cells and giant cells

Q18. Classify vascular tumors. Add a short note on Kaposi sarcoma.

Ans.

Classification of vascular tumors and tumor-like conditions:

A. Benign neoplasms

- *Hemangioma*: Capillary hemangioma, cavernous hemangioma, pyogenic granuloma
- *Lymphangioma*: Simple (capillary) lymphangioma, cavernous lymphangioma (cystic hygroma)
- Glomus tumor
- *Vascular ectasias*: Nevus flammeus, spider telangiectasia, hereditary hemorrhagic telangiectasis
- Reactive vascular proliferations: Bacillary angiomatosis

B. Intermediate-grade neoplasms

○ Kaposi sarcoma
○ Hemangioendothelioma

C. Malignant neoplasm

○ Angiosarcoma
○ Hemangiopericytoma

Kaposi sarcoma (KS)

○ Caused by human herpesvirus 8 (HHV8)
○ Associated with acquired immunodeficiency syndrome (AIDS)

Four forms:

1. *Classic KS:*

   ○ Presents as multiple red-purple skin plaques or nodules
   ○ Seen in the distal lower extremities
   ○ Tumors are asymptomatic and remain localized to the skin and subcutaneous tissue

2. *Endemic African KS*

   ○ Involves lymph nodes
   ○ Poor prognosis

3. *Transplant-associated KS*

   ○ Increased risk in solid organ transplant recipient patients
   ○ Involves lymph nodes, mucosa, and viscera

4. *AIDS-associated (epidemic) KS*

   ○ Represents the most common HIV-related malignancy
   ○ Involves lymph nodes and disseminates widely to viscera

Pathogenesis

○ KS lesions are infected by human herpesvirus 8 (HHV8), also known as Kaposi sarcoma herpesvirus

Morphology

Cutaneous lesions in classic KS progresses through three stages:

a. Patches:

   ○ Red-purple macules localized to the distal lower extremities
   ○ **Microscopy**: Dilated irregular endothelial cell-lined vascular spaces with interspersed lymphocytes, plasma cells, and macrophages

b. Plaques
- From patches, the lesions become larger, violaceous, **raised plaques**
- **Microscopy:** Dermis is composed of dilated vascular channels lined by plump spindle-shaped cells

c. Nodules

Microscopy
- Composed of sheets of plump, proliferating spindle cells surrounding small blood vessels in the dermis
- Characterized by marked hemorrhage, hemosiderin pigment, and mononuclear inflammatory cells
- Mitotic figures are common

12

White Blood Cells Disorder and Lymph Nodes

Q1. Enumerate the causes of eosinophilia.

Ans.

Causes of increased eosinophil count:
- Allergic disorders such as asthma, hay fever
- Parasitic infestations
- Drug reaction
- Malignancies (Hodgkin disease)
- Autoimmune disorders (pemphigus, dermatitis herpetiformis)
- Vasculitis

Q2. Write a note on leukemoid reaction.

Ans.

Leukemoid reactions
- Presence of a large number of immature granulocytes in the blood, mimicking myeloid leukemia
- More common in children
- Seen in severe infection, hemolysis or in malignancies

Q3. Write a note on agranulocytosis.

Ans.

Agranulocytosis
- Clinically significant reduction in neutrophils
- Leads to increase susceptibility of bacterial and fungal infections
- Serious infections are most likely when the neutrophil count falls below 500 per mm^3
- Most common cause is **drug toxicity,** e.g. alkylating agents, antimetabolites

Q4. Classify non-Hodgkin lymphoma.

Ans.

Non-Hodgkin lymphoma

A. Peripheral B-cell neoplasms

○ Chronic lymphocytic leukemia/Small lymphocytic lymphoma
○ Extranodal marginal zone lymphoma
○ Mantle cell lymphoma
○ Follicular lymphoma
○ Marginal zone lymphoma
○ Hairy cell leukemia
○ Plasmacytoma/plasma cell myeloma
○ Diffuse large B-cell lymphoma
○ Burkitt lymphoma

B. Peripheral T cell and NK-cell neoplasms

○ Mycosis fungoides/Sézary syndrome
○ Anaplastic large cell lymphoma
○ Angioimmunoblastic T cell lymphoma
○ Enteropathy-associated T cell lymphoma
○ Panniculitis-like T cell lymphoma
○ Hepatosplenic γδT cell lymphoma
○ Adult T cell leukemia/lymphoma
○ Extranodal NK/T cell lymphoma
○ NK-cell leukemia

C. Precursor B-cell neoplasms

○ B-cell acute lymphoblastic leukemia/lymphoma (B-ALL)

D. Precursor T cell neoplasms

○ T cell acute lymphoblastic leukemia/lymphoma (T-ALL)

Q5. Discuss acute lymphoblastic lymphoma in relation to its pathogenesis, morphology and prognosis.

Ans.

Acute lymphoblastic lymphoma (ALL)

Pathogenesis

○ 90% of ALLs have hyperploidy (>50 chromosomes)
○ T cell ALLs show gain-of-function mutations in NOTCH1

- ○ B-cell ALLs show loss-of-function mutations in PAX5 or balanced t(12;21) translocation
- ○ Mutations lead to maturation arrest of lymphoid cells with immature lymphoid cell proliferation

Morphology
- ○ **Bone marrow:** Hypercellular and packed with lymphoblasts
- ○ Tumor cells have scant basophilic cytoplasm with nuclei larger than those of small lymphocytes, stippled nuclear chromatin with convolutions in the nuclear membrane
- ○ Lymphoblasts are periodic acid–Schiff (PAS) positive, and myeloperoxidase negative

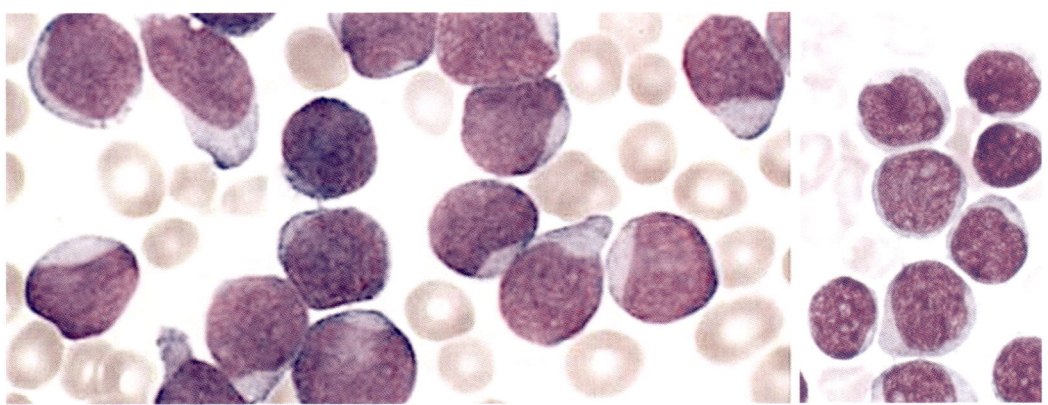

Fig. 12.1: Lymphoblasts in acute lymphoblastic leukemia

Prognosis

Worse prognostic factors
- ○ Age < 2 years
- ○ Presentation in adolescence or adulthood
- ○ High tumor burden (peripheral blood blast count greater than 100,000/mm^3)

Favorable prognostic factors
- ○ Age between 2 and 10 years
- ○ Low white cell count
- ○ Hyperdiploidy, trisomy of chromosomes 4, 7, and 10, and the presence of t(12;21)

Q6. Write a note on chronic lymphocytic leukemia.

Ans.

Chronic lymphocytic leukemia/small lymphocytic lymphoma
- ○ Most common leukemia affecting adults
- ○ In CLL, lypmhocytosis is present at the time of making diagnosis (absolute lymphocyte count) is >5000 per mm^3
- ○ **CLL**—leukemic presentation, **SLL**—localized disease
- ○ Median age at diagnosis is 60 years
- ○ M:F:: 2 : 1

Morphology
- Diffuse effacement of lymph nodes by an infiltrate of predominantly small lymphocytes

Proliferation centers
- Admixed are variable numbers of larger activated lymphocytes that form loose aggregates
- Are pathognomonic for CLL/SLL

Peripheral Smear
- A large number of small round lymphocytes with scant cytoplasm
- Smudge cells: Disrupted cells, while making smears

Immunophenotype
- Tumor cells express: CD19, CD20 (Pan B-cell markers), CD5 and CD23 positive

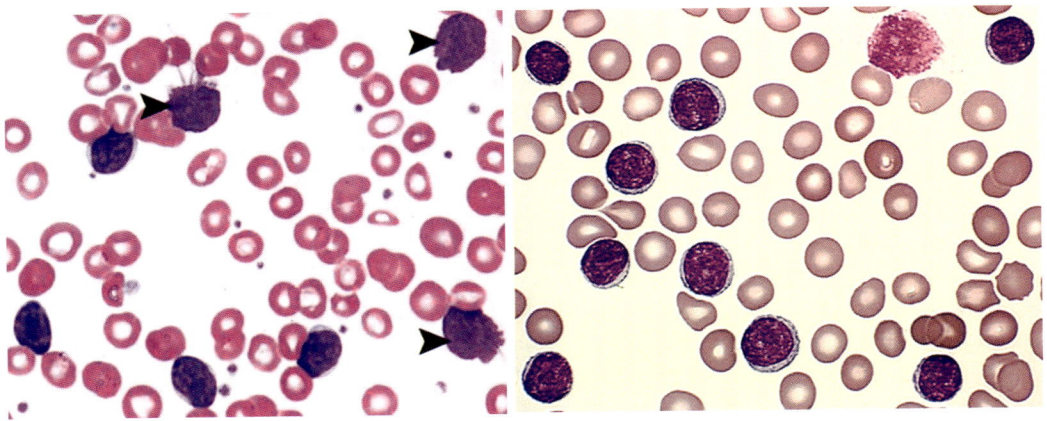

Fig. 12.2: Chronic lymphocytic leukemia with smudge cells (arrowheads)

Clinical features
- Easy fatigability, weight loss, anorexia
- Generalized lymphadenopathy and hepatosplenomegaly
- Hypogammaglobulinemia, which predisposes to infections
- Autoimmune hemolytic anemia (due to auto-antibody production by B-cells)

Q7. Write a note on Burkitt's lymphoma.

Ans.

Burkitt's Lymphoma

Three types:

1. African (endemic) Burkitt lymphoma:
- Young children, most commonly involves—**mandible**
- Abdominal viscera – kidneys, ovaries, and adrenal glands can be involved

2. **Sporadic (non-endemic) Burkitt lymphoma**:
   ○ In developing countries, affects children and young adults
   ○ Presents as mass involving the **ileocecum** and **peritoneum**
3. **HIV associated Burkitt lymphoma**:
   ○ Involves lymph nodes, brain, bone marrow, liver and GIT

Pathogenesis
○ All three types of Burkitt's lymphomas are associated with EBV infection
○ Associated with **increased MYC expression**

Increased MYC expression occurs due to either of the following translocations:
○ t(8;14): IgH locus on chromosome 14 and MYC on chromosome 8
○ t(2;8): Igκ on chromosome 2 and MYC on chromosome 8
○ t(8;22): Igλ on chromosome 22 and MYC on chromosome 8

Morphology
○ Diffuse infiltrate of lymphoid cells with round to ovoid nuclei, coarse chromatin, several nucleoli and moderate amount of cytoplasm
○ Tumor exhibits a high mitotic index and contains numerous apoptotic cells
○ Nuclear remnants of these apoptotic cells are phagocytosed by benign macrophages
○ These phagocytes have abundant clear cytoplasm, creating a characteristic "starry sky" pattern

Immunophenotype
○ Tumor cells express CD19, CD20, CD10, BCL6

Note
○ Burkitt lymphoma is very aggressive but responds well to intensive chemotherapy
○ Most children and young adults can be cured

Q8. Write a note on diagnostic criteria of symptomatic multiple myeloma.
Ans.
Diagnostic criteria of symptomatic multiple myeloma:
a. **M-protein in serum or urine**
   — No levels of serum proteins are included. However, most cases have IgG >3 g/dl, IgA >2.5 g/dl or >1 gm/24 hr of urine light chain
b. **Bone marrow clonal plasma cells or plasmacytoma**
   — No minimal level is designated; however, monoclonal plasma cells exceed 10% of nucleated cells
c. **Related organ or tissue impairment** (CRAB: Hypercalcemia, renal insufficiency, anemia, bone lesions)
   — Manifestations of end organ damage are the most important criteria of symptomatic myeloma

Q9. A 70-year-old woman admitted with worsening anemia and pathological fracture of the humerus had an ESR of 120 mm in 1 hour. Her peripheral smear showed increased rouleaux formation. X-ray of the skull showed multiple punched out osteolytic lesions.

a. What is the most probable diagnosis? Write briefly on the etiopathogenesis of this disease.

b. Describe the bone marrow changes of this disease.

c. Enumerate the diagnostic criteria of symptomatic multiple myeloma.

Ans.

Diagnosis: Multiple myeloma

Pathogenesis of **multiple myeloma:**
a. Translocations of **Ig heavy-chain (IgH) gene** on chromosome **14q32** with
   ○ **Cyclin D1** on chromosome 11q13
   ○ **Cyclin D3** on chromosome 6p21
b. Deletions of **chromosome 17p**
c. Mutations involving **NF-κB pathway** and rearrangements involving **MYC**

Morphology
○ Pathological fractures are seen in vertebral column followed by ribs, skull, pelvis, femur, clavicle, and scapula (in descending order)
○ Bone lesions appear radiographically as **punched-out defects**, measuring 1 to 4 cm in diameter
○ Marrow contains an increased number of plasma cells, comprising **>30%** of the cellularity
○ Plasma cells have an eccentrically placed nucleus with perinuclear clearing (due to prominent Golgi apparatus)

Other cells which can be seen in marrow
○ Flame cells with fiery red cytoplasm
○ Mott cells with multiple grape-like cytoplasmic droplets
○ Russell bodies: Intra-cytoplasmic globular inclusions
○ Dutcher bodies: Intra-nuclear inclusions

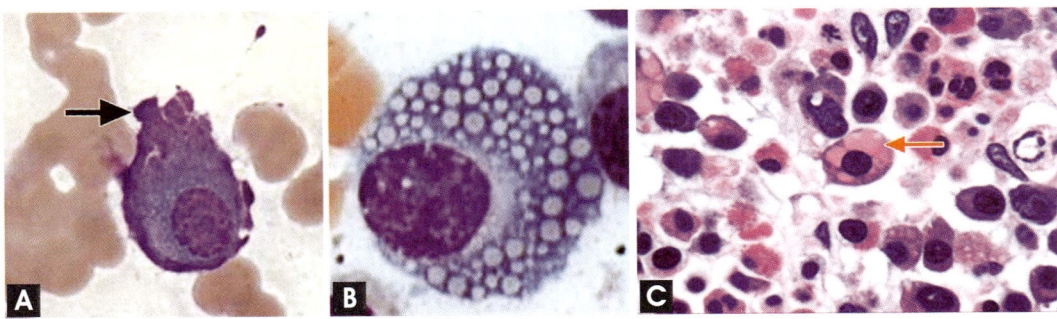

Fig. 12.3: Cells and inclusions in multiple myeloma: (A) Flame cell; (B) Mott cell; (C) Russell body

Peripheral Smear
- **Rouleaux formation** can be seen
- **Plasma cell leukemia:** Tumor cells (plasma cells) appear in peripheral blood

Diagnostic criteria of symptomatic multiple myeloma: (already discussed above)

a. M-protein in serum or urine:
  — No levels of serum proteins are included. However, most cases have IgG >3 g/dl, IgA >2.5 g/dl or >1 gm/24 hr of urine light chain

b. Bone marrow clonal plasma cells or plasmacytoma:
  — No minimal level is designated; however, monoclonal plasma cells exceed 10% of nucleated cells

c. Related organ or tissue impairment (CRAB: Hypercalcemia, renal insufficiency, anemia, bone lesions)
  — Manifestations of end organ damage are the most important criteria of symptomatic myeloma

Q10. Discuss the pathognomonic features of hairy cell leukemia.

Ans.

Hairy cell leukemia
- Affects middle-aged males, M:F::5:1

Pathogenesis
- Associated with BRAF mutations in >90% of cases

Clinical features
- Massive splenomegaly is the most common finding
- Hepatomegaly and lymphadenopathy
- Pancytopenia due to marrow infiltration and splenic sequestration
- Infections—increased incidence of **atypical mycobacterial infections**
- Excellent prognosis

Morphology
- Leukemic cells have fine hair-like projections that are best recognized under phase-contrast microscope
- **Peripheral smear:** Hairy cells has round, oblong, or reniform nuclei and moderate amounts of pale blue cytoplasm with thread-like or bleb-like extensions
- **Bone marrow aspirate:** Tumor cells are enmeshed in reticulin fibrils, which results in **dry tap**

Immunophenotype
- Hairy cell leukemias express pan-B-cell markers CD19 and CD20, and distinctive markers, such as CD11c, CD25, CD103, and annexin A1

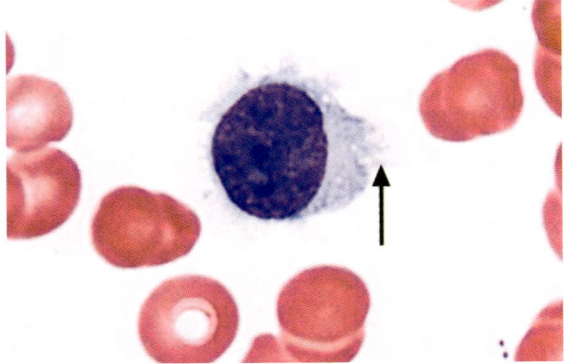

Fig. 12.4: Hairy cell in a peripheral smear

Q11. Discuss in detail the classification, molecular pathogenesis and morphology of Hodgkin lymphoma and its types.

Ans.

WHO classification recognizes five subtypes of *Hodgkin lymphoma (HL)*

A. Classical types:

1. Nodular sclerosis
2. Mixed cellularity
3. Lymphocyte-rich
4. Lymphocyte depletion

B. Lymphocyte predominance type

Pathogenesis of Hodgkin lymphoma

1. **NF-κB gets activated by one of the following mechanisms:**
   a. Due to EBV infection, which turns on genes that promote lymphocyte survival and proliferation
   b. EBV-positive tumor cells express latent membrane protein-1 (LMP-1), that up-regulate NF-κB
   c. Reed-Sternberg cells show gains in REL proto-oncogene on chromosome 2p, which leads to increase in NF-κB activity
2. Florid accumulation of reactive cells in the tissues involved by classical HL occurs in response to a wide variety of cytokines (e.g. IL-5, IL-10, and M-CSF), chemokines (e.g. eotaxin), and other factors (e.g. immunomodulatory factor galectin-1)

Morphology

- Diagnostic Reed-Sternberg (RS) cells are large cells (45 μm in diameter) with abundant cytoplasm and single or multiple nucleus
- Nucleus of RS cell has a large inclusion-like nucleolus about the size of a small lymphocyte (5 to 7 μm in diameter)
- RS cells undergo a peculiar form of cell death in which the cells shrink and become pyknotic, a process described as "mummification"

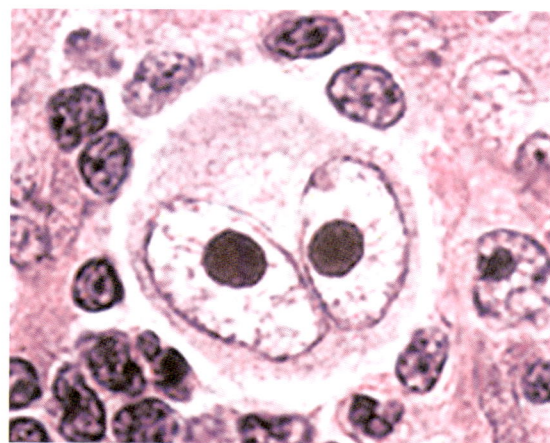

Fig. 12.5: Reed-Sternberg cell with bi-lobed nucleus (owl's eye appearance)

Variants

a. Nodular sclerosis type

- Most common form of Hodgkin lymphoma
- Deposition of collagen in bands is seen that divide the involved lymph nodes into circumscribed nodules
- Characterized by the presence of lacunar cell variant of Reed-Sternberg cell
- **Lacunar cells:** Folded or multilobated nucleus, that lies within a open space, which is an artifact created by disruption of the cytoplasm during tissue sectioning, leaving the nucleus sitting in an empty hole (a lacuna)
- Reed-Sternberg cells are found in a polymorphous background of T cells, eosinophils, plasma cells, and macrophages
- Excellent prognosis

b. Mixed-cellularity type

- Diffuse effacement of lymph nodes, with a cell population comprising of T cells, eosinophils, plasma cells and macrophages admixed with Reed-Sternberg cells
- Mononuclear variants of RS cell are seen
- Mononuclear RS cell: Contains a single nucleus with a large inclusion-like nucleolus

c. Lymphocyte rich variant

d. Lymphocyte depleted variant

Note:

- All above four mentioned subtypes are associated with EBV infection
- Immunophenotype of HL cells show PAX-5 (B-cell transcription factor), CD15, and CD30 positivity

e. Lymphocyte predominance variant:

- Effacement of lymph node by nodular infiltrate of small lymphocytes admixed with L&H (lymphocytic and histiocytic) variants of RS cells (popcorn cells)

○ **Lymphohistiocytic variants (L&H) cells** have infolded nuclear membranes, small nucleoli, fine chromatin, and abundant pale cytoplasm
○ L&H variant cells express **CD20 and BCL6**, and are negative for CD15 and CD30
○ Not associated with EBV infection

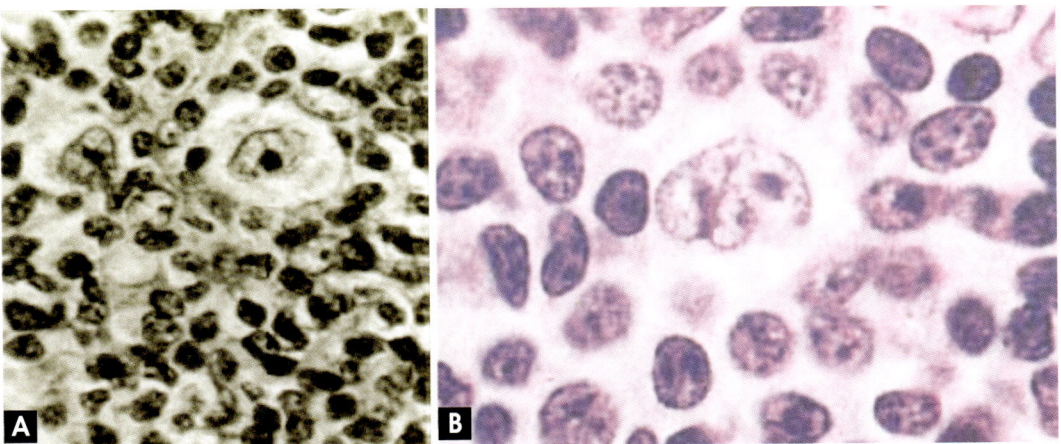

Fig. 12.6 A and B: (A) Lacunar cell; (B) Popcorn cell

Q12. Differentiate between Hodgkin lymphoma and non-Hodgkin lymphoma.

Ans.

Hodgkin lymphoma	Non-Hodgkin lymphoma
Localised to a single axial group of lymph nodes (cervical, mediastinal, para-aortic)	Involvement of multiple peripheral lymph nodes
Orderly spread by contiguity	Non-contiguous spread
Mesenteric and Waldeyer rings are rarely involved	Mesenteric and Waldeyer rings are frequently involved
Extranodal presentation is rare	Extranodal presentation is common

Q13. What is mycosis fungoides?

Ans.

Mycosis fungoides

○ Tumor comprising of CD4+ helper T cells, which shows infiltration of the epidermis and upper dermis by neoplastic T cells
○ Neoplastic T cells appear cerebriform due to marked infolding of the nuclear membranes
○ Involvement of the skin is manifested as generalized exfoliative erythroderma

Sézary syndrome

○ When the tumor cells (Sézary cells) invade the peripheral blood
○ Leukemia comprising of Sézary cells, with characteristic cerebriform nuclei

Q14. Classify acute myeloid leukemia. Describe molecular pathogenesis, lab investigations and clinical features of acute myeloid leukemia.

Ans.

WHO classification acute myeloid leukemia:

1. AML with genetic aberrations:

- ○ AML with t(8;21)
- ○ AML with inv (16)
- ○ AML with t(15;17)
- ○ AML with t(11q23)

2. AML with MDS-like features

3. AML, therapy-related

4. AML, not otherwise specified

- ○ AML, minimally differentiated
- ○ AML without maturation
- ○ AML with myelocytic maturation
- ○ AML with myelomonocytic maturation
- ○ AML with monocytic maturation
- ○ AML with erythroid maturation
- ○ AML with megakaryocytic maturation

Pathogenesis:

- ○ t(8;21) and inv (16) lead to formation of fusion gene products, which block the maturation of myeloid cells
- ○ AML with t(15;17) (acute promyelocytic leukemia) leads to formation of PML-RAR (retinoic acid receptor-α) fusion gene product, which interferes with the terminal differentiation of granulocytes
- ○ Patients with PLM-RARα mutations can be treated with either all-trans retinoic acid or arsenic trioxide

Lab diagnosis and morphology

- ○ Number of leukemic cells in blood vary from more than $100,000/mm^3$ to $10,000/mm^3$
- ○ Diagnosis of AML is based on the presence of at least 20% myeloid blasts
- ○ Myeloblasts have delicate nuclear chromatin, two to four nucleoli, and more voluminous cytoplasm than lymphoblasts
- ○ Auer rods, distinctive needle-like azurophilic granules, are present in AML with the t(15;17) (acute promyelocytic leukemia)
- ○ Monoblasts have folded or lobulated nuclei, and lack Auer rods
- ○ In AML, if blasts show megakaryocytic differentiation, marrow can show accompanying fibrosis

○ **Aleukemic leukemia:** Blasts are entirely absent from the blood
○ Bone marrow examination is essential to exclude acute leukemia in pancytopenic patients

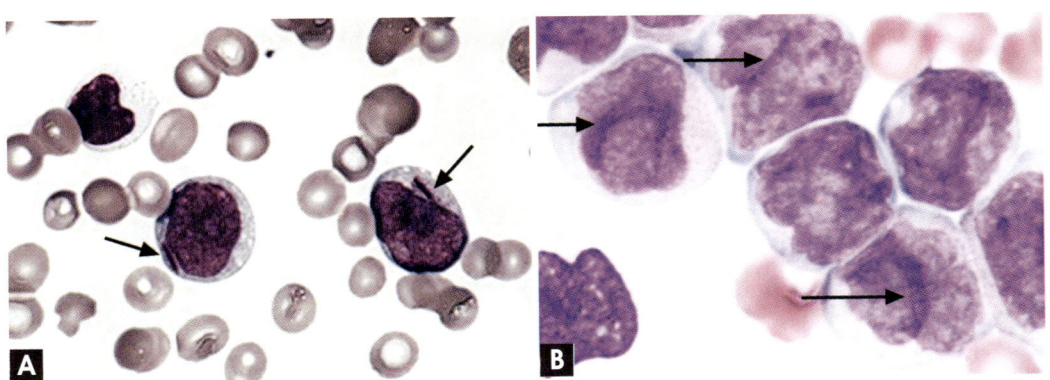

Fig. 12.7A and B: (A) Myeloblasts with Auer rods; (B) Monoblasts

Note:
○ Myeloid precursors show MPO positivity
○ Monoblasts, promonocytes show non-specific esterase (NSE) positivity
○ Erythroid precursors show PAS positivity

Clinical features
○ Anemia, neutropenia, and thrombocytopenia, leading to fatigue, fever, and spontaneous mucosal and cutaneous bleeding
○ Procoagulants and fibrinolytic factors released in AML with t(15;17), exacerbate the bleeding tendency
○ Tumors with monocytic differentiation often infiltrate the skin (leukemia cutis) and the gingiva
○ Occasionally, it presents as a localized soft-tissue mass known as myeloid sarcoma or chloroma

Q15. Write a note on myelodysplastic syndromes.

Ans.
Myelodysplastic syndromes
○ Clonal stem cell disorders characterized by maturation defects
○ Associated with ineffective hematopoiesis and a high risk of transformation to AML
○ Two types—primary (idiopathic) or secondary to drug or radiation therapy (t-MDS)

Classification of MDS (WHO)
1. Refractory anemia
2. Refractory anemia with ring sideroblasts
3. Refractory cytopenia with multilineage dysplasia (RCMD)
4. Refractory anemia with excess blasts-1 (RAEB-1)

5. Refractory anemia with excess blasts-2 (RAEB-2)
6. MDS-U (unclassified)
7. MDS with isolated del (5q) deletion

Morphology of MDS:
Bone marrow examination:

○ **Cellularity**: Hypercellular marrow, can be normocellular or hypocellular
○ **Characteristic finding:** Dyspoises affecting the erythroid, granulocytic, monocytic, and megakaryocytic lineages
a. **Erythroid series:**
   ○ **Ring sideroblasts** (erythroblasts with iron-laden perinuclear granules seen on Prussian blue-stain)
   ○ **Megaloblastoid maturation** and **nuclear budding** abnormalities
b. **Myeloid lineage:**
   ○ Neutrophils contain decreased numbers of secondary granules, toxic granulations and/or Döhle bodies
   ○ **Pseudo-Pelger-Hüet cells:** Neutrophils with only two nuclear lobes
c. **Megakaryocytic lineage:**
   ○ **Pawn ball megakaryocytes:** Megakaryocytes with multiple separate nuclei

Note:

○ Myeloblasts can be increased but comprises <20% of marrow cellularity

Q16. Describe chronic myeloid leukemia in relation to its peripheral smear, bone marrow findings and clinical outcome.

Ans.

Chronic myelogenous leukemia:

○ Characteristic feature is BCR-ABL gene fusion product derived from portions of the BCR gene on chromosome 22 and the ABL gene on chromosome 9
○ BCR-ABL is created by (9;22) translocation (the so-called Philadelphia [Ph] chromosome)
○ BCR-ABL gene product leads to increase proliferation of granulocytic and megakaryocytic precursors with their release into the blood

Morphology

a. **Chronic phase**
   Bone marrow
   ○ Markedly hypercellular marrow with increased numbers of granulocytic precursors
   ○ Megakaryocytes are also increased and usually include small, dysplastic forms
   ○ Erythroid progenitors are present in normal or mildly decreased numbers
   ○ **Sea-blue histiocytes:** Presence of scattered macrophages with abundant wrinkled, green-blue cytoplasm

Peripheral smear in chronic phase
- Leukocytosis >100,000 cells/mm^3
- Consists predominantly of band forms and myelocytes admixed with neutrophils, eosinophils, and basophils
- < 10% blasts are seen
- Elevated platelet count
- Splenomegaly, as a result of extramedullary hematopoiesis

b. Accelerated phase
- Persistent or increasing WBC count or increasing splenomegaly
- Persistent thrombocytosis
- Persistent thrombocytopenia
- 20% or more basophils
- 10–19% myeloblasts in the blood or bone marrow

c. Blast phase
- Blasts are equivalent to or greater than 20%
- Extramedullary blast proliferation
- In 70% of cases, blast lineage is myeloid and in 20–30% cases blasts are of lymphoid lineage

Clinical features
- Anemia
- Splenomegaly (producing dragging sensation in abdomen or acute onset left upper quadrant pain due to splenic infarction)
- Treatment: BCR-ABL inhibitors

Q17. Write the diagnostic criteria of polycythemia vera.

Ans.
Diagnostic criteria for polycythemia vera (PV)

a. Major criteria
- Hemoglobin >18.5 gm/dl in men, 16.5 gm/dl in women
- Presence of JAK2 V617F mutation

b. Minor criteria
- Bone marrow biopsy showing hypercellularity for age with increase in all three cell lines (panmyelosis)
- Serum erythropoietin levels below the reference range for normal
- Endogenous erythroid colony formation *in vitro*

Note:
For diagnosis PV, 2 major and 1 minor criteria are required.

Q18. Write a note on primary myelofibrosis.

Ans.
Primary myelofibrosis
WHO criteria for primary myelofibrosis:

Major:

1. Presence of megakaryocytic proliferation and atypia, accompanied by fibrosis
2. Not meeting WHO criteria for polycythemia vera, CML, MDS
3. Demonstration of JAK2 V617F mutation or other clonal marker

Minor:

1. Leucoerythroblastosis
2. Increase in serum lactate dehydrogenase levels
3. Anemia
4. Splenomegaly

Note:

For diagnosing, all 3 major and 2 minor criteria should be fulfilled

Morphology:

Bone marrow (early/cellular phase):

○ Marrow is hypercellular due to increase in maturing cells of all lineages
○ Erythroid and granulocytic precursors appear normal, but megakaryocytes are large, dysplastic, and abnormally clustered

Bone marrow (late phase):

○ Hypocellular and diffusely fibrotic
○ Clusters of atypical megakaryocytes with "cloud-like" nuclei are seen
○ Hematopoietic elements are found within dilated sinusoids

Q19. Discuss Langerhans cell histiocytosis.

Ans.

Langerhans cell histiocytosis (LCH)

○ Histiocytosis means proliferation of dendritic cells or macrophages
○ In LCH, there occurs proliferation of immature dendritic cells, i.e. Langerhans cell
○ Most commonly associated with BRAF mutation

Can present as:

a. Letterer-Siwe disease

   ○ Age <2 years
   ○ Cutaneous lesions (seborrheic eruptions), over the front and back of trunk and on scalp
   ○ Hepatosplenomegaly, lymphadenopathy, pulmonary lesions, destructive osteolytic bone lesions
   ○ Anemia, thrombocytopenia and recurrent infections due to bone marrow infiltration
   ○ Rapidly fatal

b. Eosinophilic granuloma

   ○ Arises within the medullary cavities of bones, most commonly the calvarium, ribs, and femur

◯ **Hand-Schüller-Christian triad:** Calvarial bone defects, exophthalmos and diabetes insipidus (due to involvement of pituitary stalk)

◯ Eosinophils make a prominent component of the infiltrate

◯ Spontaneous remission and good prognosis

c. Pulmonary Langerhans cell histiocytosis

◯ Adult smokers, due to reactive proliferations of Langerhans cells

◯ May regress spontaneously upon cessation of smoking

Morphology

◯ Langerhans cells have abundant, vacuolated cytoplasm and vesicular nuclei containing linear grooves or folds

◯ Tumor cells express **S-100 and CD1a**

Electron microscopy

◯ Presence of Birbeck granules in the cytoplasm is characteristic

◯ Birbeck granules are rod shaped with dilated terminal ends producing a tennis racket-like appearance, and contains the protein **langerin**

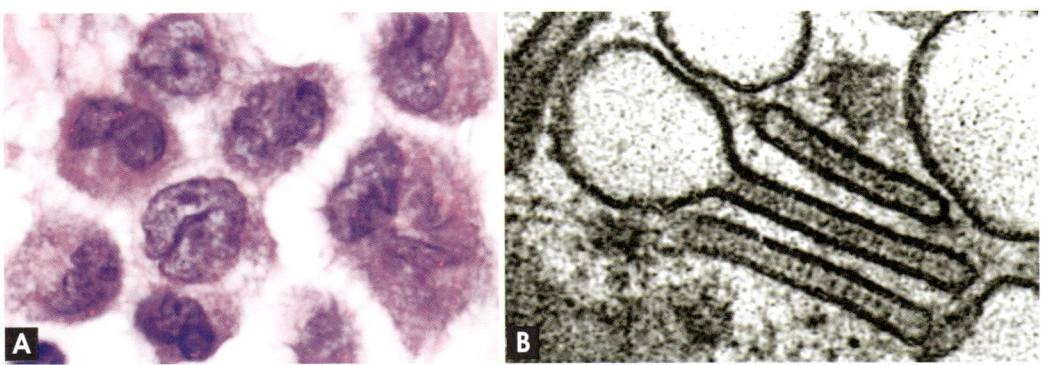

Fig. 12.8A and B: (A) Langerhans cell in LCH; (B) Birbeck granules on EM

Red Blood Cells and Bleeding Disorders

Q1. Define anemia.

Ans.

Definition: Reduction of total circulating red cell mass below normal limits

Diagnosis is made by:
a. Reduction in hematocrit or
b. Reduction in hemoglobin concentration of blood to the levels that are below the normal range

Note

Normal hemoglobin (gm/dl) levels in adults:
13.6–17.2 in males
12.0–15.0 in females

Q2. Write classification of anemia.

Ans.

Mechanism	Specific examples
1. Blood loss	Trauma, GIT lesions
2. Increased red cell destruction (hemolysis)	
a. Inherited genetic defects	Hereditary spherocytosis, hereditary elliptocytosis, G6PD deficiency, pyruvate kinase deficiency
b. Hemoglobin abnormalities	Thalassemia, sickle cell anemia
c. Acquired genetic defect: Deficiency of phosphatidylinositol-linked glycoproteins	Paroxysmal nocturnal hemoglobinuria
d. Antibody-mediated destruction	Hemolytic disease of newborn, transfusion reactions, drug induced, autoimmune disorders
e. Microangiopathic hemolytic anemia	Hemolytic uremic syndrome, disseminated intravascular coagulation, thrombotic thrombocytopenic purpura
f. Infections	Malaria

Contd.

Contd.

3. Decreased red cell production

a. Inherited genetic defects	Fanconi anemia
b. Nutritional deficiency	Vitamin B_{12}, folate and iron deficiency anemia
c. Erythropoietin deficiency	Renal failure, anemia of chronic disease
d. Inflammation mediated iron sequestration	Anemia of chronic disease
e. Hematopoietic neoplasms	Acute leukemia, myelodysplasia, myeloproliferative neoplasms
f. Space occupying marrow lesions	Metastatic neoplasms, granulomatous disease

Q3. Write a note on red cell indices.

Ans.

Red cell indices

○ **Mean cell volume (MCV):** Average volume of a red cell expressed in femtoliters (fl)

○ **Mean cell hemoglobin (MCH):** Average content (mass) of hemoglobin per red cell, expressed in picograms

○ **Mean cell hemoglobin concentration (MCHC):** Average concentration of hemoglobin in a given volume of packed red cells, expressed in grams per deciliter

○ **Red cell distribution width (RDW):** Coefficient of variation of red cell volume

Adult reference ranges

Measurement	
Mean cell volume (fl)	82–96
Mean cell hemoglobin (pg)	27–33
Mean cell hemoglobin concentration (gm/dl)	33–37
Red cell distribution width	11.5–14.5

Q4. Enumerate the differences between extravascular hemolysis and intra-vascular hemolysis.

Ans.

	Extravascular hemolysis	Intravascular hemolysis
S. methemalbumin	–ve	+ve
Plasma hemoglobin	–ve	+ve
Serum bilirubin (unconjugated)	++	+
Serum LDH	+	++
Urine hemoglobin	–ve	+ve
Urine hemosiderin	–ve	+ve
Tissue iron	Increased	Decreased
Examples	Thalassemia, sickle cell anemia	PNH, G6PD deficiency

Q5. Discuss the pathogenesis and morphology of hereditary spherocytosis.

Ans.

Hereditary spherocytosis (HS)

○ Autosomal dominant disorder
○ Characterized by inherited defects in red cell membrane
○ Red cells become spherical, less deformable, vulnerable to splenic sequestration and destruction

Pathogenesis

○ RBC membrane components include α-spectrin, β-spectrin, ankyrin, band 4.2 or band 3
○ Mutations most commonly affect ankyrin, band 3, spectrin, or band 4.2
○ Mutations result in loss of red cell membrane fragments
○ Due to loss of membrane, the red cell assumes the smallest possible diameter for a given volume, i.e. a sphere

Consequences of the mutation

○ Spherocytes are less deformable than normal RBCs and are trapped in the splenic cords, where they are phagocytosed by macrophages
○ Young HS red cells are normal in shape, but as they age, they shed the membrane fragments
○ Life span of the affected red cells is decreased to 10 to 20 days from the normal 120 days

Morphology

○ **Spherocytes:** Smears show small, hyperchromic RBCs, that lack the central zone of pallor
○ Increased reticulocyte count, marrow erythroid hyperplasia, hemosiderosis and mild jaundice
○ Cholelithiasis (pigment stones)
○ Moderate splenomegaly (congestion of splenic cords and increased phagocytes)

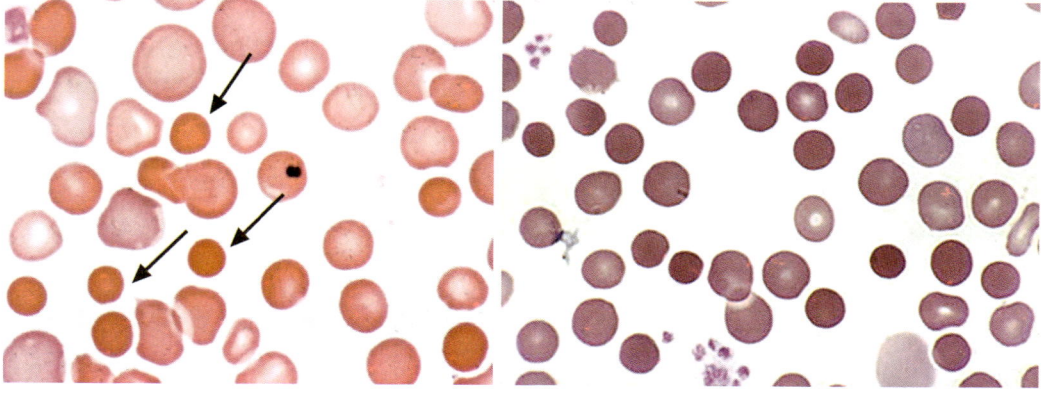

Fig. 13.1: Spherocytes (arrow) in peripheral smear in hereditary spherocytosis

Q6. Write a note on pathogenesis of sickle cell anemia and the factors affecting the rate of sickling.

Ans.

Pathogenesis

○ Oxygenated hemoglobin is a free flowing liquid

○ Deoxygenated hemoglobin (HbS) gets converted from free flowing liquid into a viscous gel followed by long needle like fibers, producing a sickle or holly-leaf shape

Factors affecting rate of sickling

a. Interaction of HbS with the other types of hemoglobin in the cell:

○ **HbA:** More HbA levels, less sickling (seen in sickle cell trait)

○ **HbF:** Inhibits the polymerization of HbS, hence infants do not become symptomatic till 6 months of age

○ **HbSC disease:** Individuals with both HbS and HbC have symptomatic sickling disorder (termed HbSC disease)

b. Mean cell hemoglobin concentration (MCHC):

○ Conditions which increase MCHC increase sickling, e.g. dehydration

○ Conditions which reduce MCHC reduces sickling

c. Intracellular pH:

○ Decrease in pH, reduces the oxygen affinity of hemoglobin (as a result fraction of deoxygenated HbS increases), thereby increasing the sickling

d. Transit time of red cells through microvascular beds:

○ Sickling is confined to the vessel walls where the blood flow is slow (slow transit time)

○ Blood flow is sluggish in normal spleen, bone marrow, and inflamed vascular beds which are prominently affected in sickle cell disease

Q7. Discuss the morphology, lab investigations, clinical features and treatment of sickle cell anemia.

Ans.

Morphology

Peripheral smear

○ Increased numbers of irreversibly sickled cells, target cells, Howell-Jolly bodies (small nuclear remnants) are present

○ Increased reticulocyte count

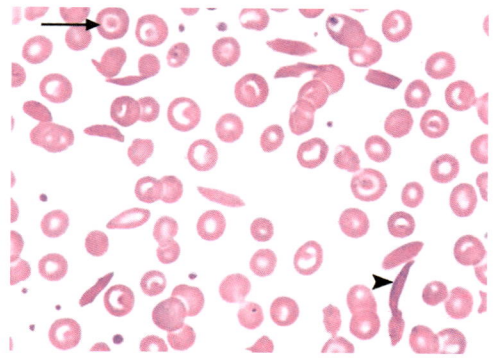

Fig. 13.2: Sickle red cells (arrowhead) and target cells (arrow) in peripheral smear

Bone marrow

○ Hypercellular with compensatory erythroid hyperplasia

○ Expansion of the marrow leads to bone resorption and secondary new bone formation, resulting in prominent cheekbones and "crew-cut" appearance of the skull on X-ray

Spleen

○ Enlarged due to red pulp congestion, caused by trapping of sickled red cells in cords and sinuses

○ Due to chronic erythrostasis, spleen becomes infarcted, fibrosed and shrunken, over time, resulting in **autosplenectomy**

Infarction

○ Can be seen in bones, brain, kidney, liver, retina, and pulmonary vessels

○ Vascular stagnation in subcutaneous tissues leads to leg ulcers

Clinical features

1. **Vaso-occlusive crises (pain crises):**

   a. Painful bone crises: Dactylitis of the bones of hands or feet

   b. Acute chest syndrome: Vaso-occlusive crisis involving the lungs, presents as fever, cough, chest pain, and pulmonary infiltrates

   c. Priapism may lead to erectile dysfunction

   d. Stroke and retinopathy

2. **Sequestration crises:**

   ○ Massive entrapment of sickle red cells leads to rapid splenic enlargement, hypovolemia, and shock

   ○ *Pneumococcus pneumoniae* and *Haemophilus influenzae* septicemia are common due to poor splenic function

3. **Aplastic crises**: Occur due to infection of red cell progenitors by parvovirus B19

Lab diagnosis

○ **Sickling test:** Sickling can be induced by mixing a blood sample (with HbS) with an oxygen consuming reagent, such as sodium metabisulfite

○ **Hemoglobin electrophoresis:** To demonstrate the presence of HbS and exclude other sickle syndromes, such as HbSC disease

Treatment

○ Hydroxyurea
   a. Increases red cell HbF levels
   b. An anti-inflammatory effect (inhibition of leukocyte production)
○ Hematopoietic stem cell transplantation offers a chance for cure

Q8. Discuss in detail the pathogenesis, morphology and clinical course of beta thalassemia major.

Ans.

β-Thalassemia

○ β-globin gene is located on chromosome 11
○ Caused by mutations that diminish the synthesis of β-globin chains

Molecular pathogenesis

○ β0 mutations (absent β-globin synthesis)
○ β+ mutation (reduced β-globin synthesis)

Mutation includes

○ **Splicing mutations:** Most common cause of β+ thalassemia, resulting in absent/reduced production of β-globin mRNA

○ **Promoter region mutations:** Mutations reduce transcription of proteins, leading to β+-thalassemia

○ **Chain terminator mutations:** Most common cause of β0-thalassemia, due to frame shift mutations or introduction of stop codons

Morphology

a. Peripheral smear

○ Marked variation in size (anisocytosis) and shape (poikilocytosis) of RBCs, microcytosis, and hypochromia

○ Target cells (hemoglobin collects in the center of the cell), basophilic stippling, and fragmented red cells can be seen

○ Reticulocyte count is elevated

○ Nucleated red cell precursors (normoblasts) are seen in the peripheral blood

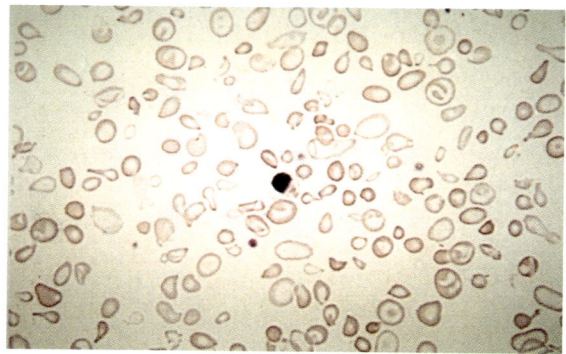

Fig. 13.3: Target cells, microcytes, anisopoikilocytosis, nRBC in peripheral smear of thalassemia patient

b. Bone marrow and spleen

- Expansion of the hematopoietically active marrow
- Bones of the face and skull erodes the existing cortical bone with resultant new bone formation, giving rise to a "crew cut" appearance on X-ray studies
- Spleen weighs as much as 1500 gm

c. Hemosiderosis or secondary hemochromatosis is seen in every patient

Clinical course

- Children, who are not treated with blood transfusion, die at an early age
- Hepatosplenomegaly is seen, due to extramedullary hematopoiesis
- Cardiac disease (important cause of death) due to progressive iron overload and secondary hemochromatosis
- Patients receiving multiple blood transfusions must be treated with iron chelators to prevent hemochromatosis
- Hematopoietic stem cell transplantation can offer cure

Q9. Write a brief note on Bart's hemoglobin.

Ans.

Bart's Hemoglobin

- Results in hydrops fetalis
- Most severe form of α-thalassemia, which is caused by deletion of all four α-globin genes
- In fetus, excess γ-globin chains form tetramers **(Bart's Hemoglobin)**
- Bart's Hemoglobin has a high affinity for oxygen and hence oxygen delivery to the tissues is markedly decreased
- Fetus shows severe pallor, generalized edema, massive hepatosplenomegaly, similar to that seen in hemolytic disease of newborn
- Signs of fetal distress become evident by third trimester of pregnancy

Q10. Write a note on paroxysmal nocturnal hemoglobinuria.

Ans.

Paroxysmal nocturnal hemoglobinuria **(PNH)**

- **Hemolytic anemia** caused by an **acquired genetic defect**
- Results due to **acquired mutations** in the **phosphatidylinositol glycan complementation group A gene (PIGA)**
- PIGA mutation leads to deficiency of **GPI-linked proteins**
- **Increased susceptibility** of all **three cell lines** (RBC, WBC, platelets) to **complement mediated lysis**

PNH cells are deficient in three GPI-linked proteins

- Decay accelerating factor, or CD55
- Membrane inhibitor of reactive lysis, or CD59
- C8 binding protein

CD59 is a potent inhibitor of C3 convertase that prevents the spontaneous activation of alternative complement pathway

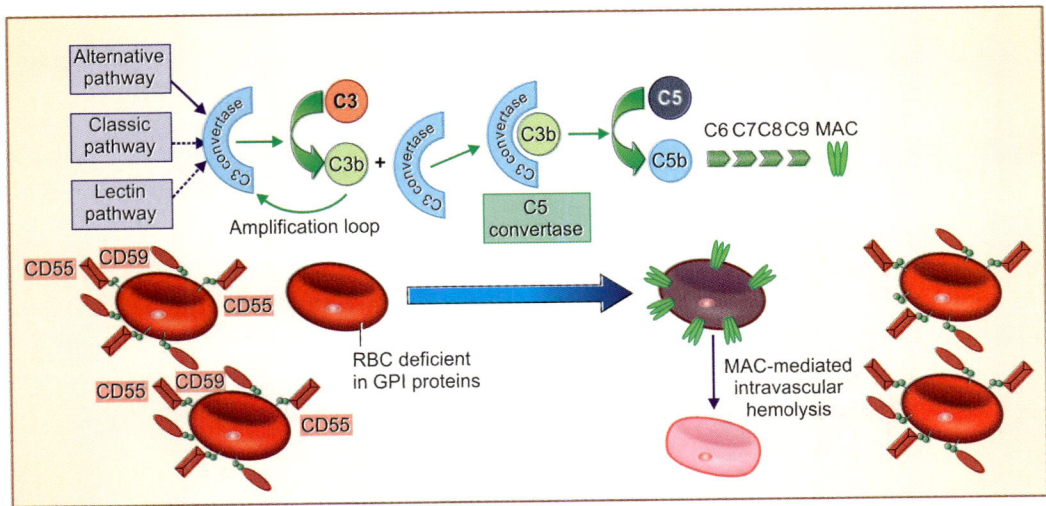

Fig. 13.4: Pathogenesis of PNH

CD59, CD55 deficient RBCs are destroyed by membrane attack complex with resultant hemolysis.

Clinical features and lab diagnosis

- Manifests as intravascular hemolysis (due to activation of membrane attack complex)
- Hemolysis is paroxysmal and nocturnal (due to decrease in blood pH during sleep, which increases blood complement activity)
- Thrombosis is the most common cause of death in individuals with PNH
- 5 to 10% of patients develop **acute myeloid leukemia** or **myelodysplastic syndrome**
- PNH is diagnosed by **flow cytometry**

Treatment
- ○ Eculizumab (monoclonal antibody) prevents the conversion of C5 to C5a
- ○ Monoclonal antibody reduces the risk of hemolysis and thrombosis
- ○ Complication: C5 inhibitor therapy leads to an increased risk of serious or fatal meningococcal infections

Q11. Classify immune hemolytic anemia.

Ans.

Classification of immunohemolytic anemias
1. Warm antibody type (IgG antibodies active at 37°C)
   - ○ Primary (idiopathic)
   - ○ Secondary: Autoimmune disorders (systemic lupus erythematosus, RA), drugs (penicillin, cephalosporins, α-methyldopa), lymphoid neoplasms (CLL), malignant lymphoma, Hodgkin disease, multiple myeloma, thymoma, AML
2. Cold agglutinin type (IgM antibodies active below 37°C)
   - ○ Acute: Mycoplasma infection, infectious mononucleosis
   - ○ Chronic: Idiopathic, lymphoid neoplasm
3. **Cold hemolysin type** (IgG antibodies active below 37°C)

Q12. Write a note on Coombs' test.

Ans.

Diagnosis of immunohemolytic anemia requires the detection of antibodies and/or complement on the RBCs of the patient

a. *Direct Coombs' anti-globulin test*
   - ○ Patient's red cells are mixed with polyspecific anti-human globulin (AHG) (anti-IgG and anti-complement)
   - ○ If either immunoglobulin or complement is present on the surface of the red cells, antibodies cause agglutination, appreciated visually as clumping

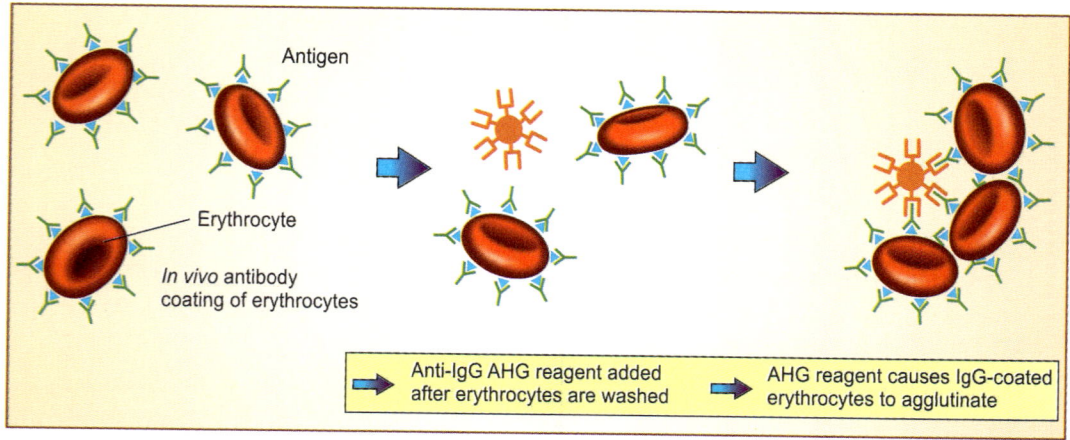

Fig. 13.5: Direct antiglobulin test

b. *Indirect Coombs' anti-globulin test*

- Used to detect antibodies in the patients serum
- Positive indirect Coombs' test indicates alloimmunization (immunization to the antigens from another individual) and/or presence of autoantibody in the patients serum

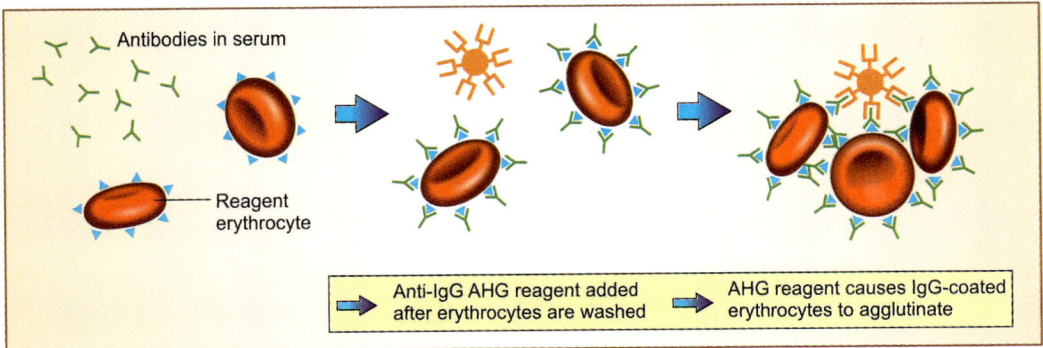

Fig. 13.6: Indirect antiglobulin test

Q13. Write a note on hemolytic uremic syndrome.

Ans.

Hemolytic uremic syndrome (HUS)

- HUS is associated with microangiopathic hemolytic anemia and thrombocytopenia with acute renal failure (in children)
- Intravascular thrombi cause microangiopathic hemolytic anemia
- Thrombocytopenia occurs due to consumption of platelets
- Coagulation tests in HUS will be normal

Types

a. "Typical" HUS

- Associated with infectious gastroenteritis caused by *Escherichia coli strain* O157:H7, which elaborates Shiga-like toxin
- Toxin, absorbed from the inflamed gastrointestinal mucosa, enters into the circulation and results in altered endothelial cell function leading to platelet activation and aggregation

b. "Atypical" HUS

- Defects in complement factor H, factor I or membrane cofactor protein (CD46) which prevent excessive activation of alternative complement pathway
- **Pathogenesis:** Excessive complement activation, results in endothelial injury and platelet aggregation

Q14. Write a note on osmotic fragility.

Ans.

Osmotic fragility test

- ○ Red cells are suspended in decreasing concentrations of hypotonic saline solutions to check their ability to withstand osmotic stress
- ○ In hypotonic solutions, water enters RBCs causing cellular swelling followed by cell lysis

Increased osmotic fragility is seen in:

- ○ Hereditary spherocytosis
- ○ Autoimmune hemolytic anemia
- ○ Hemolytic diseases of newborn

Decreased osmotic fragility is seen in:

- ○ Iron deficiency anemia
- ○ Thalassemia
- ○ Asplenia
- ○ Liver disease
- ○ Reticulocytosis
- ○ Presence of HbS and HbC

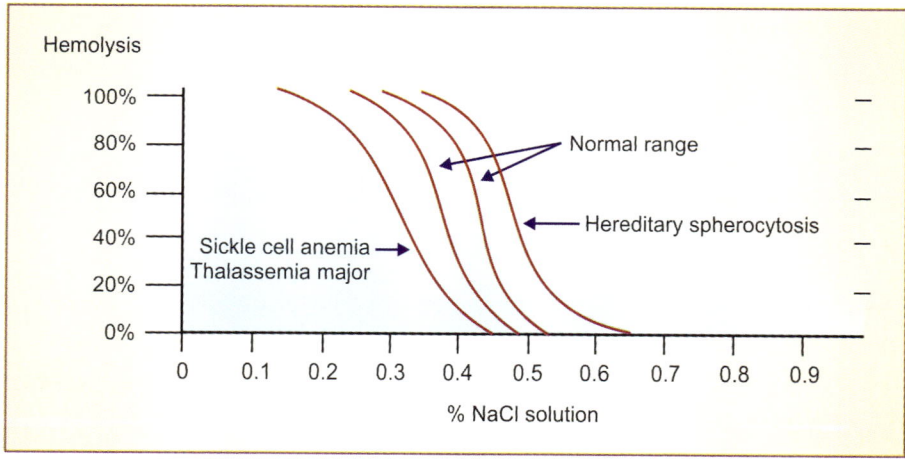

Fig. 13.7: Osmotic fragility graph with examples

Q15. List the causes of megaloblastic anemia. Discuss about the pathogenesis, morphology and bone marrow picture of megaloblastic anemia.

Ans.

Megaloblastic anemia occurs due to vitamin B_{12} deficiency or folic acid deficiency.

1. Causes of vitamin B_{12} deficiency

a. *Decreased intake*

- ○ Inadequate diet, vegetarianism

   b. *Impaired absorption*
   - **Intrinsic factor deficiency:** Pernicious anemia, gastrectomy
   - Malabsorption states
   c. *Diffuse intestinal disease (e.g. lymphoma, systemic sclerosis)*
   d. *Ileal resection, ileitis*
2. Causes of folic acid deficiency
   a. Decreased intake
   - Inadequate diet, alcoholism, infancy
   - Impaired absorption
   - Malabsorption states
   - Anticonvulsants
   - Oral contraceptives
   b. Increased requirement
   - Pregnancy, infancy, disseminated cancer, markedly increased hematopoiesis
   c. Impaired utilization
   - Folic acid antagonists
   d. Unresponsive to vitamin B_{12} or folic acid therapy
   - DNA synthesis and/or folate metabolism inhibitors (e.g. methotrexate)

Pathogenesis
- Occurs due to impairment of DNA synthesis

Morphology

Peripheral smear
- Macro-ovalocytes: RBCs are oval and macrocytic, larger than normal, lack central pallor of normal red cells
- Marked variation in the size (anisocytosis) and shape (poikilocytosis) of red cells
- Reticulocyte count is low
- In severe anemia, nucleated red cell progenitors appear in the blood
- Neutrophils are larger than normal (macropolymorphonuclear) and show nuclear hypersegmentation (having five or more nuclear lobules)

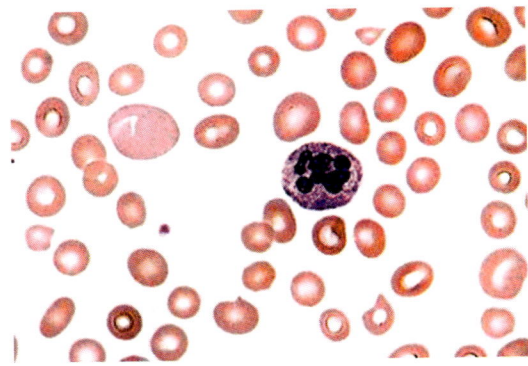

Fig. 13.8: Peripheral smear showing a macrocyte and hypersegmented neutrophil

Bone marrow

○ Markedly hypercellular marrow with increased hematopoietic precursors
○ Megaloblastic changes are detected at all stages of erythroid development
○ Megaloblasts are large nucleated erythroid precursors whose nuclear maturation lags behind cytoplasmic maturation
○ Nucleus of megaloblast contains loose, open seive-like chromatin
○ Nuclear-to-cytoplasmic asynchrony: Nuclear maturation is delayed, cytoplasmic maturation proceed at a normal pace
○ Granulocytic precursors show dysmaturation in the form of giant metamyelocytes and band forms
○ Megakaryocytes are abnormally large with bizarre multilobated nuclei

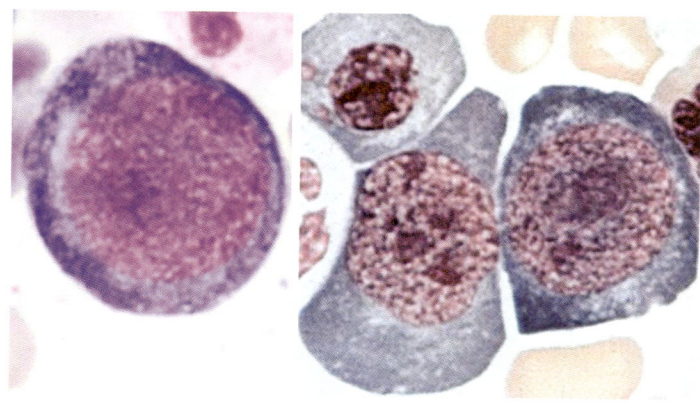

Fig. 13.9: Megaloblasts with sieve-like chromatin in megaloblastic anemia

Q16. Discuss the etiopathogenesis, peripheral smear and bone marrow findings in iron deficiency anemia.

Ans.

Etiology:

Iron deficiency anemia results from:

○ Dietary lack of iron
○ Impaired absorption
○ Increased requirement
○ Chronic blood loss

Note:

○ 1 mg of iron must be absorbed from the diet everyday
○ Daily iron requirement: 7 to 10 mg for adult men, 7 to 20 mg for adult women (only 10% to 15% of ingested iron is absorbed)
○ Absorption of inorganic iron is increased by ascorbic acid, citric acid, amino acids, sugars and is inhibited by tannates (found in tea), carbonates, oxalates, and phosphates

Peripheral smear
- RBCs appear small (microcytic) and pale (hypochromic) with zone of pallor in RBC being enlarged
- In severe iron deficiency anemia, hemoglobin may be seen only in narrow peripheral rim
- Poikilocytosis in the form of small, elongated red cells (pencil cells) can be seen

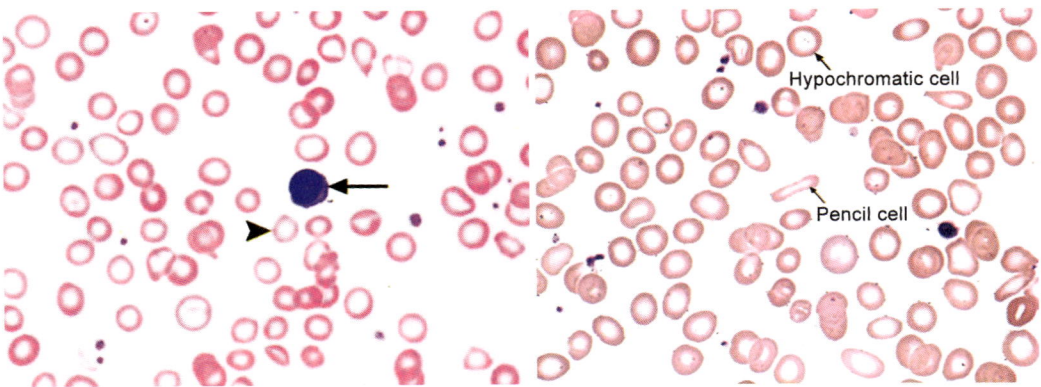

Fig. 13.10: Microcyte (small-sized RBC, compared to lymphocyte)

Bone marrow
- Mild to moderate increase in erythroid progenitors
- Prussian blue stain on bone marrow aspirate smear shows disappearance of stainable iron from the macrophages

Q17. Write a note on anemia of chronic disease.

Ans.

Anemia of chronic disease (ACD)
- Red cell production is impaired due to chronic diseases that produce systemic inflammation

Causes
- Osteomyelitis, bacterial endocarditis, lung abscess
- Immune disorders, such as rheumatoid arthritis
- Neoplasms: Carcinomas of the lung and breast and Hodgkin lymphoma

Mechanism
- Inflammatory mediators, i.e. IL-6, stimulates the hepatic hepcidin production
- Hepcidin inhibits ferroportin in macrophages and reduces the transfer of iron from storage pool to the developing erythroid precursors in the bone marrow
- Other mechanism: Cytokine mediated inhibition of erythropoietin production

Peripheral smear
- RBCs are normocytic and normochromic or microcytic and hypochromic

How to differentiate anemia of chronic disease from iron deficiency anemia?
- Bone marrow: Shows presence of increased storage iron in marrow macrophages and presence of sideroblasts
- High serum ferritin levels

Q18. Write etiology and morphology of bone marrow in aplastic anemia.

Ans.

Aplastic anemia
- Characterized by chronic primary hematopoietic failure and pancytopenia

Causes
- **Drugs:** Alkylating agents, antimetabolites, benzene, chloramphenicol, penicillamine, carbamazepine
- **Physical agents:** Irradiation, viral infections, hepatitis, cytomegalovirus, Epstein-Barr virus infection, herpes zoster (varicella zoster)
- **Inherited:** Fanconi anemia, telomerase defects

Morphology
- Markedly hypocellular bone marrow, devoid of hematopoietic cells
- Marrow shows fat cells, fibrous stroma, scattered lymphocytes, plasma cells
- Marrow aspirates give a "dry tap"
- Aplasia is best appreciated in marrow biopsies

Q19. Enumerate the entities comprising of Fanconi anemia.

Ans.

Fanconi anemia:
- Autosomal recessive disorder

Cause
- Occurs due to defects in multiprotein complex (required for DNA repair)

Comprises:
- Congenital anomalies (hypoplasia of kidney and spleen with bone anomalies, which most commonly involve the thumbs or radius bone)
- Hypoplastic bone marrow

Q20. Write a note on Bernard-Soulier syndrome.

Ans.

Bernard-Soulier syndrome
- Bleeding due to defective platelet adhesion to sub-endothelial matrix
- Due to deficiency of platelet membrane glycoprotein complex Ib-IXa, a receptor for vWF
- Gp Ib-IXa is essential for normal platelet adhesion to the sub-endothelial extracellular matrix
- Also known: Deficiency of GpIIb/IIIa results in defective platelet aggregation, a disorder termed Glanzmann thrombasthenia.

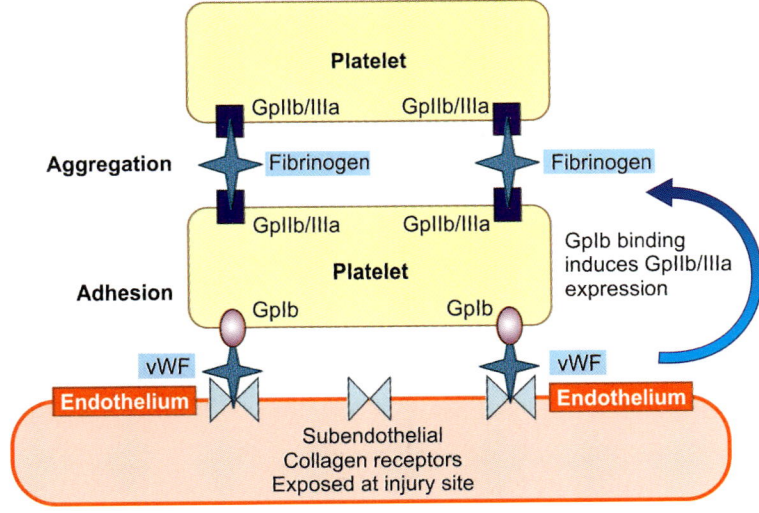

Fig. 13.11: Role of GpIb and GpIIb in platelet adhesions and aggregation

Q21. Mention the function of prothrombin time assay.

Ans.

Prothrombin time (PT) assay

- Assesses the function of the proteins in the extrinsic pathway (factors VII, X, V, II, and fibrinogen)

Q22. Write a note on von Willebrand's disease.

Ans.

von Willebrand disease

- Most common inherited bleeding disorder of humans
- Clinical features: Spontaneous bleeding from mucous membranes (e.g. epistaxis), excessive bleeding from wounds, or menorrhagia

Type 1 vWD

- Autosomal dominant disorder
- Quantitative defects in vWF
- Most common type, leads to mild disease

Type 2 vWD

- Autosomal dominant disorder
- Characterized by qualitative defects in vWF

Type 3 vWD

- Autosomal recessive disorder
- Quantitative defects in vWF
- Associated with very low levels of vWF and severe clinical manifestations

Q23. Write a note on hemophilia A.

Ans.

Hemophilia A (factor VIII deficiency)

○ Inherited as X-linked recessive trait
○ Caused by mutations in factor VIII
○ Most common hereditary disease associated with life-threatening bleeding
○ Affects males and homozygous females
○ Patients with 6% to 50% of normal factor VIII levels have mild disease
○ Patients with 2% to 5% of normal factor VIII levels have moderately severe disease
○ Patients with < 1% of normal factor VIII levels have severe disease and spontaneous hemorrhages into joints (hemarthrosis) is common
○ Petechiae are characteristically absent
○ Patients have prolonged PTT and a normal PT (due to abnormality of intrinsic coagulation pathway)
○ Hemophilia A is treated with infusions of recombinant factor VIII

Hemophilia B (Christmas disease, factor IX deficiency):

○ Inherited as X-linked recessive trait
○ PTT is prolonged and the PT is normal
○ Treatment: Infusions of recombinant factor IX

Q24. Write a note on the pathogenesis of disseminated intravascular coagulation.

Ans.

Disseminated intravascular coagulation (DIC)

○ Thrombohemorrhagic disorder characterized by excessive activation of coagulation pathway with formation of thrombi in the microvasculature throughout the body
○ Cause: Due to systemic activation of thrombin

Two major mechanisms that trigger DIC

○ Release of tissue factor (procoagulant) into the circulation
○ Widespread injury to the endothelial cells

a. Sources of tissue factor

○ Placenta in obstetric complications
○ Tissues injured by trauma or burns
○ Mucus released from adenocarcinomas

b. Endothelial injury can be seen

○ In sepsis: TNF acts as a mediator of endothelial injury
○ In systemic lupus erythematosus due to deposition of antigen–antibody complexes
○ Following heat stroke, burns
○ Following meningococci, rickettsiae infections

Consequences of DIC
- Widespread deposition of fibrin
- Hemorrhagic diathesis

Q25. Define thrombocytopenia. Write causes of thrombocytopenia.

Ans.
- Reference range of platelets: **1,50,000–4,50,000/μL**
- **Thrombocytopenia:** When platelet count is **less than 100,000 platelets/μL**

Causes of thrombocytopenia
a. Decreased platelet production
  Selective impairment of platelet production:
  - Drug-induced: Alcohol, thiazides, cytotoxic drugs
  - Infections: Measles, human immunodeficiency virus (HIV)
  Nutritional deficiencies:
  - Vitamin B_{12} and folate deficiency (megaloblastic anemia)
  Bone marrow failure:
  - Aplastic anemia
  Bone marrow replacement:
  - Leukemia, disseminated cancer, granulomatous disease
  Ineffective hematopoiesis:
  - Myelodysplastic syndromes
b. Decreased platelet survival
  Immunologic destruction:
  Primary autoimmune
  —Chronic immune thrombocytopenic purpura
  —Acute immune thrombocytopenic purpura
  Secondary autoimmune
  —Systemic lupus erythematosus, B-cell lymphoid neoplasms
  —Alloimmune: Post-transfusion and neonatal
  —Drug-associated: Quinidine, heparin, sulfa compounds
  —Infections: HIV, infectious mononucleosis (transient, mild), dengue fever
  Non-immunologic destruction:
  —Disseminated intravascular coagulation
c. Sequestration
  —Hypersplenism
d. Dilution
  —Transfusions

Q26. Write a note on idiopathic thrombocytopenic purpura.

Ans.
Acute immune thrombocytopenic purpura
- Affects children and disease is self-limited (disease resolves in 6 months)

○ Symptoms appear 1 to 2 weeks after self-limited viral illness which triggers the development of auto-antibodies

○ Glucocorticoids are given only if the thrombocytopenia is severe

Chronic immune thrombocytopenic purpura (ITP)

Pathogenesis

○ Auto-antibodies directed against platelet membrane glycoprotein IIb-IIIa or Ib-IX, and are of IgG type

Morphology

a. Spleen

   ○ Normal in size

   ○ Congestion of sinusoids with enlargement of splenic follicles, associated with prominent reactive germinal centers

b. Bone marrow

   ○ To rule out other causes of thrombocytopenia

   ○ Increased number of megakaryocytes, with large, non-lobulated, single nuclei

c. Blood

   ○ Peripheral blood reveals abnormally large platelets

Clinical features

○ Most commonly in women less than 40 years of age

○ Female-to-male ratio is 3 : 1

○ Petechiae: Cutaneous bleeding (pinpoint hemorrhage) which when confluent, can give rise to ecchymoses

○ Easy bruising, nosebleeds, bleeding from the gums, melena, hematuria, or excessive menstrual flow

○ Subarachnoid hemorrhage and intracerebral hemorrhage

○ Splenomegaly and lymphadenopathy are uncommon

○ PT and APTT are normal

Treatment

○ Glucocorticoids (inhibit phagocyte function)

○ Splenectomy normalizes the platelet count (in individuals with severe thrombocytopenia)

○ Intravenous immunoglobulin or anti-CD20 antibody (rituximab) is effective in patients who relapse after splenectomy

Q27. Write a note on complications of blood transfusion.

Ans.

Complications of blood transfusion

a. Febrile non-hemolytic reaction

   ○ Most common complication

   ○ Patient presents as fever and chills, mild dyspnea

   ○ Occurs within 6 hours of a transfusion of red cells or platelets

b. **Allergic drug reactions**
c. **Hemolytic reactions**
   - **Acute hemolytic reactions:** Due to preformed IgM antibodies against donor RBCs
   - **Delayed hemolytic reactions:** Caused by antibodies that recognize red cell antigens that the recipient was sensitized to previously, for example, through a prior blood transfusion
d. **Transfusion-related acute lung injury (TRALI)**
   - Severe, frequently fatal complication in which factors in a transfused blood product trigger the activation of neutrophils in the lung microvasculature
e. **Infectious complications**
   - HIV, hepatitis C, hepatitis B, malaria and syphilis
   - Transmission of these diseases has now decreased, due to donor screening for these infections

Q28. What is hematocrit?

Ans.

Hematocrit or packed cell volume
- Volume occupied by red blood cells when a sample of anticoagulated blood is centrifuged
- Indicates relative proportion of red cells to plasma

Uses
- Detection of presence and absence of anemia or polycythemia
- For estimation of red cell indices

Methods of estimation
- Wintrobe method
- Microhematocrit method

Q29. Write bone marrow changes in lead poisoning.

Ans

Peripheral smear
- Microcytic, hypochromic anemia
- Accompanied by mild hemolysis
- Punctate basophilic stippling of red cells

Bone marrow
- Ring sideroblasts
- Red cell precursors with iron-laden mitochondria, detected by Prussian blue stain

Q30. Write a note on Bence Jones proteins.

Ans.

Bence Jones proteins
- Monoclonal immunoglobulin light chains, synthesized by neoplastic plasma cells
- Excess production of these chains are seen in multiple myeloma and primary amyloidosis

○ Because of their low molecular weight, these are excreted in urine
○ When urine sample is heated, Bence Jones proteins precipitate at temperatures between 40° and 60°C, and the precipitate disappears on heating up to 85°–100°C, and when cooled, there is reappearance of the precipitate.
○ Investigation of choice for its detection in urine is protein electrophoresis

Q31. What is leucocyte alkaline phosphatase scoring?

Ans.

Leucocyte alkaline phosphate (LAP) score

○ It is used in patients with elevated WBC to differentiate reactive leucocytosis from chronic myelogenous leukemia
○ Reduced LAP score is seen in CML, aplastic anemia, pernicious anemia
○ Elevated LAP score is also seen in leukemoid reaction (or reactive leucocytosis), myelofibrosis, essential thrombocytosis and polycythemia vera

14

Lung

Q1. Write a note on Atelectasis.

Ans.

Atelectasis: Defined as collapse of the lung

Major types:

- **Resorption atelectasis:** Due to complete obstruction of the airway. Causes include bronchial asthma, chronic bronchitis, bronchiectasis, aspiration of foreign bodies and fragments of bronchial tumors
- **Compression atelectasis:** Due to fluid or air in pleural cavity
- **Contraction atelectasis:** Pulmonary or pleural fibrosis prevents full lung expansion

Note

- Resorption and compression types are reversible

Q2. Write about causes, pathogenesis and morphology of acute respiratory distress syndrome (ARDS).

Ans.

Acute respiratory distress syndrome (diffuse alveolar damage)

- Characterized by abrupt onset of significant hypoxemia and bilateral pulmonary infiltrates in the absence of cardiac failure
- Acute respiratory distress syndrome (ARDS) is a manifestation of severe acute lung injury (ALI)
- Most common causes: Sepsis, pulmonary infections, gastric aspiration, mechanical trauma

Pathogenesis

Following events occur in sequence leading to alveolar damage:

1. Endothelial activation
2. Adhesion and extravasation of neutrophils
3. Accumulation of intra-alveolar fluid and formation of hyaline membranes
4. Resolution of injury with resultant fibrosis of alveolar walls

Morphology
- ○ Lungs are heavy, firm, red and boggy and shows congestion, interstitial and intra-alveolar edema, inflammation, **fibrin** deposition, and **diffuse alveolar damage**
- ○ Alveolar walls are lined with waxy **hyaline membranes**

Q3. Write a note on etiopathogenesis and histological types of emphysema.

Ans.

Emphysema
- ○ Characterized by irreversible enlargement of the airspaces distal to the terminal bronchiole, accompanied by destruction of their walls without obvious fibrosis
- ○ Four major types:
  1. Centriacinar
  2. Panacinar
  3. Paraseptal
  4. Irregular

1. Centriacinar (centrilobular) emphysema
- ○ Central or proximal parts of the acini, formed by respiratory bronchioles, are affected, whereas distal alveoli are spared
- ○ Lesions are more common and severe in the upper lobes
- ○ Seen in heavy smokers, in association with chronic bronchitis (COPD)

2. Panacinar (panlobular) emphysema
- ○ Acini are uniformly enlarged and involves alveolar duct and alveolus
- ○ More common in the lower zones, most severe at the bases
- ○ Associated with α_1-antitrypsin deficiency

3. Distal acinar (paraseptal) emphysema
- ○ Distal acinus is involved, severe in the upper half of the lungs
- ○ Multiple, continuous, enlarged airspaces
- ○ Cause of spontaneous pneumothorax in young adults

4. Irregular emphysema
- ○ Acinus is irregularly involved, and is associated with scarring

Q4. Write a short note on chronic bronchitis.

Ans.

Chronic bronchitis
- ○ **Definition:** Persistent cough with sputum production for at least 3 months in at least 2 consecutive years, in the absence of any other identifiable cause

Pathogenesis: Exposure to tobacco smoke and dust from grain, cotton, and silica leads to:

a. Mucus hypersecretion: Associated with hypertrophy of submucosal glands in trachea and bronchi

b. Inflammation

c. Infection

Morphology
- ○ Increase in number of goblet cells and mucus gland layer hyperplasia

○ Bronchial epithelium can exhibit squamous metaplasia and dysplasia
○ **Bronchiolitis obliterans:** Marked narrowing of bronchioles due to fibrosis, which results in obliteration (in severe cases)

Reid index: (normal value: 0.4)
○ Ratio of the thickness of mucous gland layer to the thickness of the wall between the epithelium and the cartilage
○ **Increased** in chronic bronchitis

Q5. Write a short note on the pathogenesis of bronchial asthma.

Ans.

Asthma
○ Episodic bronchoconstriction due to increased airway sensitivity to a variety of stimuli; inflammation of the bronchial walls; and increased mucus secretion

Pathogenesis
1. TH2 responses, IgE and inflammation
Early reaction
a. Inhaled allergens (antigen) stimulate TH2 cells and result in IgE production
b. IgE results in eosinophil recruitment
c. On re-exposure to the antigen, there occurs cross-linking of IgE, bound to the Fc receptors on mast cells resulting in release of mast cell mediators
d. Mast cell mediators bring about bronchospasm, increased vascular permeability, mucus production, recruitment of leukocytes

Late reaction
e. Leukocytes recruited to the site and factors released from eosinophils (e.g. major basic protein, eosinophil cationic protein), damages the epithelium

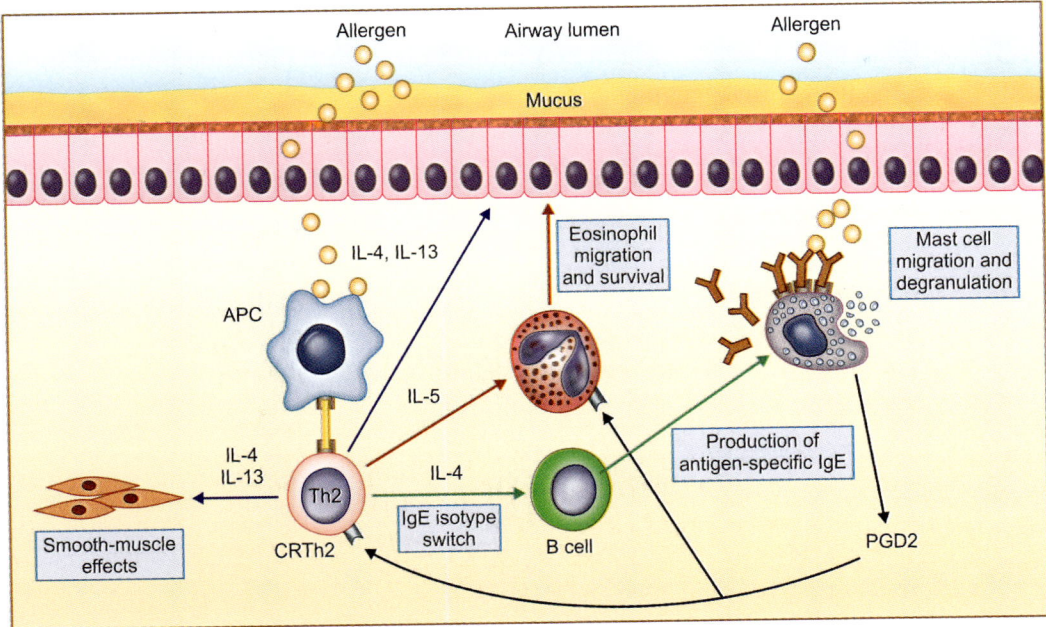

Fig. 14.1: Pathogenesis of asthma

2. **Genetic susceptibility:** Polymorphism in IL-13 gene and gene encoding ADAM33 increases the risk
3. **Environmental factors:** Allergen, smoke acts as induction factors

Morphology of asthmatic airway
○ Accumulation of mucus
○ Goblet cell hyperplasia
○ Thickened basement membrane
○ Intense chronic inflammation (eosinophils, macrophages)
○ Hypertrophy and hyperplasia of smooth muscle cells
○ Hypertrophy of submucosal glands

Q6. Discuss the causes and morphology of lung in bronchiectasis.

Ans.

Definition
○ Permanent dilation of the bronchi and bronchioles due to destruction of smooth muscle and elastic tissue by chronic necrotizing infections

Causes

a. **Congenital or hereditary conditions:** Cystic fibrosis, primary ciliary dyskinesia and Kartagener syndromes
b. **Infections:** Pneumonia
c. **Bronchial obstruction:** Tumor, foreign bodies, or mucus impaction
d. Rheumatoid arthritis, systemic lupus erythematosus, inflammatory bowel disease, COPD

Morphology
○ Affects bilateral lower lobes, and is most severe in distal bronchi and bronchioles
○ Airway dilatation is seen, and dilated bronchioles can be followed almost to the pleural surfaces
○ **Cut surface of the lung shows** dilated bronchi, which appear cystic and are filled with mucopurulent secretions

Q7. Write a note on pneumoconiosis.

Ans.

Definition: Non-neoplastic lung reaction due to the inhalation of mineral dusts encountered in the workplace

Important pneumoconiosis and their implicated causative agent

Disease	Causative agent
Anthracosis	Coal dust
Silicosis	Silica
Asbestosis	Asbestos
Farmer's lung	Moldy hay
Bagassosis	Bagasse
Byssinosis	Cotton

Q8. Discuss coal worker pneumoconiosis.

Ans.

Coal workers' pneumoconiosis

○ Caused by inhalation of coal particles

Can present as

a. Anthracosis

○ Pulmonary lesion seen in coal miners

○ Inhaled carbon pigment is engulfed by alveolar or interstitial macrophages and are deposited along the bronchi

b. Simple coal workers' pneumoconiosis

○ Characterized by coal macules (1 to 2 mm in diameter) and coal nodules

○ **Sites:** Upper lobes and upper zones of the lower lobes

c. Complicated coal workers' pneumoconiosis (progressive massive fibrosis)

○ Characterized by multiple, intensely blackened scars of 1 cm or larger

○ **Microscopy:** Lesions consist of dense collagen and pigment

Q9. Write salient features of silicosis.

Ans.

Silicosis

○ Caused by inhalation of crystalline silicon dioxide (silica)

Pathogenesis

○ Silica occurs in crystalline and amorphous forms

○ Crystalline forms (e.g. quartz) are more fibrogenic

○ After inhalation, the particles are phagocytosed by macrophages and activate inflammasome, which releases inflammatory mediators, IL-1 and IL-18.

Morphology

○ **Gross:** Nodules in upper zones of the lungs, which in chronic stages coalesce into hard, collagenous scars

○ Fibrotic lesions can also occur in the hilar lymph nodes and pleura

○ **Eggshell calcification:** Thin sheets of calcification in the lymph nodes, seen radiographically

Microscopy

○ Central area of whorled collagen fibers with peripheral zone of dust-laden macrophages

○ Nodules with polarized microscopy reveals birefringent silica particles

Note

○ Silicosis is associated with increased susceptibility to tuberculosis and lung cancer

Q10. Mention asbestos related diseases and their pathogenesis.

Ans.

Asbestos-related diseases include

○ Localized fibrous plaques, or rarely, diffuse pleural fibrosis
○ Pleural effusions
○ Parenchymal interstitial fibrosis (asbestosis)
○ Lung carcinoma
○ Mesotheliomas (pleural and peritoneal)
○ Laryngeal, ovarian and colon carcinomas
○ Increased risk for systemic autoimmune diseases and cardiovascular disease

Pathogenesis

○ **Two distinct forms:** Serpentine chrysotile (most commonly used) and Amphibole (more pathogenic)
○ After inhalation, particles are phagocytosed by macrophages, resulting in activation of inflammasome
○ Inflammasome activation brings about interstitial inflammation and fibrosis

Morphology

○ **Asbestos bodies:** Golden brown, fusiform or beaded rods with a translucent center
○ Asbestosis begins in the lower lobes and subpleurally

Pleural plaques

○ Most common manifestation of asbestos exposure
○ Well-circumscribed plaques of dense collagen
○ **Sites:** Parietal pleura and over the domes of the diaphragm

Q11. Write a note on sarcoidosis.

Ans.

Sarcoidosis

○ Systemic granulomatous disease that presents as bilateral hilar lymphadenopathy or lung involvement

Pathogenesis

○ Intra-alveolar and interstitial accumulation of CD4+ T cells, resulting in CD4/CD8 T cell ratios ranging from 5 : 1 to 15 : 1
○ Association with HLA-A1 and HLA-B8

Morphology

○ Non-necrotizing granulomas composed of aggregates of tightly clustered epithelioid macrophages, and giant cells
○ In **giant cells: Schumann bodies** (laminated concretions composed of calcium and proteins) and **stellate inclusions (asteroid bodies)** are found

Q12. Discuss lobar pneumonia.

Ans.

Lobar pneumonia

○ Consolidation of large portion of a lobe or of an entire lobe of the lung

Stages

Four stages of the inflammatory response are seen

a. Congestion
- ○ Lung is heavy, boggy, and red
- ○ Characterized by vascular engorgement, intra-alveolar fluid with a few neutrophils

b. Red hepatization
- ○ **Gross:** Affected lobe of lung is red, firm, and airless, with liver-like consistency
- ○ **Microscopy:** Alveolar spaces with exudates comprising of neutrophils, red cells, and fibrin

c. Gray hepatization
- ○ Characterized by progressive disintegration of red cells and persistence of fibrinosuppurative exudate

d. Resolution
- ○ Exudates in the intra-alveolar spaces gets broken down and is ingested by macrophages, which is either expectorated or gets organized by fibroblasts

Complications of pneumonia include

a. Abscess formation: Due to tissue destruction and necrosis

b. Empyema: Spread of infection to the pleural cavity

c. Bacteremic dissemination: To the heart valves, pericardium, brain, kidneys, spleen, or joints

Q13. Discuss the pathogenesis and morphology of lung in primary pulmonary tuberculosis.

Ans.

Pathogenesis: Involves the following steps

a. Entry of *Mycobacterium tuberculosis* bacilli into the macrophages

b. Replication of tubercle bacilli in the macrophages occurs because tubercle bacilli inhibits maturation of the phagosome and blocks the formation of phagolysosome

c. Th1 response: After 3 weeks of the initial infection, T cells transform into T-helper 1 (Th1) cells, by IL-12

d. Th1-mediated macrophage activation and killing of bacteria: Th1 cell mediates IFN-γ production and thus enables macrophages to contain *M. tuberculosis*

e. Granulomatous inflammation and tissue damage

A. Primary pulmonary tuberculosis (0–3 weeks)

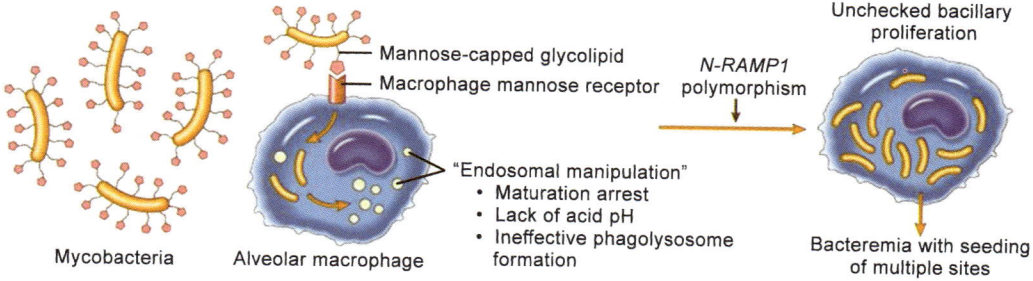

Fig. 14.2: Primary tuberculosis (1–3 weeks)

B. Primary pulmonary tuberculosis (>3 weeks)

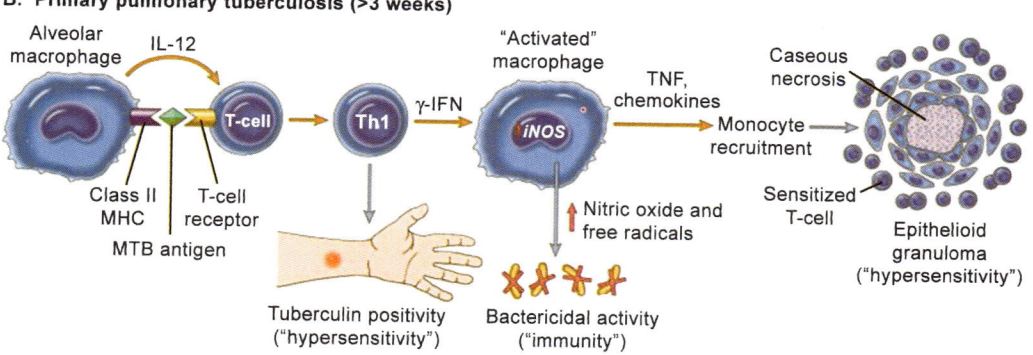

Fig. 14.2: Primary tuberculosis (>3 weeks)

Morphology of lung in primary pulmonary tuberculosis
Primary tuberculosis

- **Ghon focus**: 1 to 1.5 cm area of consolidation, with caseous necrosis in its centre
- **Ghon complex:** Combination of parenchymal lung lesion and nodal involvement
- After cell mediated immunity controls the infection, Ghon complex undergoes progressive fibrosis, resulting in radiologically detectable calcification (Ranke complex)

Microscopy

- Consolidated areas show caseation necrosis with surrounding epithelioid cell granulomas, and multinucleated Langhans giant cells

Q14. Classify bronchogenic carcinoma. Discuss the etiopathogenesis and morphology of various subtypes.
Ans.

Histologic classification of malignant epithelial lung tumors

a. Squamous cell carcinoma
b. Small cell carcinoma
c. Adenocarcinoma
d. Large cell carcinoma

e. Adenosquamous carcinoma

f. Carcinomas with pleomorphic, sarcomatoid, or sarcomatous elements

g. Carcinoid tumor

Etiology and pathogenesis

o **Tobacco smoking**

o **Industrial hazards:** Asbestos, arsenic, chromium, uranium, nickel, vinyl chloride, high-dose ionizing radiation

o **Air pollution:** Radon gas exposure increases the risk

Molecular Genetics

a. **Squamous cell carcinoma:** Chromosome 3p, 9p and 17p (TP53) deletions, amplification of FGFR1

b. **Small cell carcinoma:** Shows strongest association with smoking, p53 mutations, Rb gene deletions, chromosome 3p deletions

c. **Adenocarcinoma:** Gain-of-function mutations in EGFR, RET receptors and KRAS gene mutations

Morphology

o Adenocarcinoma arises in the periphery of lung, whereas squamous cell carcinomas arise in the central/hilar region

a. **Adenocarcinoma**

   o Patterns recognizable on histopathology: Acinar, lepidic, papillary, micropapillary, and solid, with or without mucin production

   o Are located peripherally and are smaller

   o Shows thyroid transcription factor-1 (TTF-1) positivity

   o **Microinvasive adenocarcinoma:** Tumors with a small invasive component (≤5 mm)

   o **Mucinous adenocarcinoma** can present as satellite nodules

b. **Squamous cell carcinoma**

   o Most commonly found in men and is strongly associated with smoking

   o Presence of keratinization and/or intercellular bridges

   o Keratinization may take the form of squamous pearls

   o **Precursor lesions:** Squamous metaplasia, epithelial dysplasia, carcinoma *in situ*

c. **Small cell carcinoma**

   o Arises in major bronchi or in the periphery of the lung

   o Has a strong relationship to cigarette smoking

   o Most aggressive lung tumors

   o Most commonly associated with ectopic hormone production

Microscopy

o Small cells with scant cytoplasm, ill-defined cell borders, finely granular nuclear chromatin (salt and pepper pattern), and absent or inconspicuous nucleoli

o Tumor cells are round, oval, or spindle shaped, and nuclear molding is prominent

o Mitotic count is high, with extensive necrosis

○ **Azzopardi effect:** Basophilic staining of vascular walls due to encrustation by DNA from necrotic tumor cells

○ **IHC:** Chromogranin, synaptophysin, CD57 positivity, and high levels of antiapoptotic protein BCL2 are seen in 90% of tumors

Q15. Mention paraneoplastic syndromes associated with carcinoma lung.

Ans.

Paraneoplastic syndromes

○ Hyponatremia: Due to ADH
○ Cushing syndrome: Due to ACTH
○ Lambert-Eaton syndrome
○ Hypercalcemia: Due to parathormone, parathyroid hormone-related peptide, prostaglandin E
○ Hypocalcaemia: Due to calcitonin
○ Gynecomastia: Due to gonadotropins
○ Carcinoid syndrome: Due to serotonin and bradykinin

Q16. Write a short note on mesothelioma.

Ans.

Malignant mesothelioma

○ Associated with heavy exposure to asbestos

Genetics

○ Deletion of tumor suppressor gene CDKN2A/INK4a are seen in 80% of mesotheliomas

Morphology

Gross

○ Arises from visceral or parietal pleura
○ Thick, firm, white pleural tumor tissue ensheathes the lung

Microscopy

a. **Epithelioid type**
   ○ Consists of cuboidal, columnar, or flattened cells forming tubular or papillary structures resembling adenocarcinoma
   ○ IHC: Positive for calretinin, Wilms' tumor 1 (WT-1), cytokeratin 5/6, and D2-40
b. **Sarcomatoid type**
   ○ Mesenchymal type, appears as spindle cell sarcoma
c. **Mixed (biphasic) type:** Contains both epithelioid and sarcomatoid patterns

Note

○ Fifty percent of patients die within 12 months of diagnosis

15

Head and Neck

Q1. Classify salivary gland tumors.

Ans.

Salivary gland tumors

1. Benign

- ○ Pleomorphic adenoma, Warthin tumor, oncocytoma, basal cell adenoma, ductal papilloma

2. Malignant

- ○ Mucoepidermoid carcinoma, adenocarcinoma not otherwise specified (NOS), acinic cell carcinoma, adenoid cystic carcinoma, malignant mixed tumor, squamous cell carcinomas

Q2. Write a note on adamantinoma of jaw.

Ans.

Ameloblastoma/Adamantinoma of jaw

- ○ Most common epithelial odontogenic tumors
- ○ Age group: 3–5 decades
- ○ Most common site: Mandible
- ○ X-ray demonstrates a lytic expansile lesion

Gross

- ○ Solid and cystic

Microscopy

- ○ Follicular and plexiform subtypes are most common
- ○ Follicular type: Follicles containing basaloid cells lining the basement membrane and the central portion of the follicle resembles stellate reticulum
- ○ Plexiform type: Irregular masses and cords of epithelial cells within stroma

Q3. Write a note on pleomorphic adenoma of salivary gland.

Ans.

Pleomorphic adenoma (mixed tumors)

○ Benign tumors that consist of a mixture of ductal (epithelial) and myoepithelial cells

○ Most common site is parotid gland

Risk factors

○ Radiation exposure increases the risk

○ Chromosomal rearrangements involving **PLAG1**

Morphology

Gross

○ Presents as a **rounded, encapsulated, well-demarcated masses**

○ **Cut surface:** Gray-white with myxoid like areas

Microscopy

○ **Epithelial elements** are arranged in acini, tubules, strands, or sheets of cells

○ Epithelial cells in the ducts are surrounded by myoepithelial cell layer in a background of myxoid substance

Q4. Write a note on Warthin's tumor of salivary gland.

Ans.

Warthin tumor (papillary cystadenoma lymphomatosum)

○ Arises from the parotid gland

○ Occurs more commonly in males

○ Age group: Fifth to seventh decades of life

○ 10% are multifocal and 10% are bilateral

○ **Smokers** are at increased risk of developing these tumors

Gross

○ Round encapsulated mass

○ Cut surface: It shows multiple cystic spaces containing serous or mucinous secretions

Microscopy

○ Cystic spaces are lined by a double layer of neoplastic epithelial cells resting on a dense lymphoid stroma with prominent germinal centers

○ Cystic space lumen often contains secretions

Q5. Write a note on malignant salivary gland tumors.

Ans.

Mucoepidermoid carcinomas

○ Most common **primary malignant tumor** of the salivary glands

○ Most common site: **Parotid gland** followed by minor salivary glands

Morphology
Gross
○ Circumscribed tumor, but lack well-defined capsule
○ Cut surface—solid with small, mucin-containing cysts

Microscopy
○ Tumor grows in nests, sheets and cords
○ Tumor cells are composed of mixtures of squamous cells, mucus-secreting cells and intermediate cells

Adenoid Cystic Carcinoma
○ Most common site—**minor salivary glands (palate)**
○ Can show perineural invasion

Gross
○ Small, poorly encapsulated, infiltrative lesions

Microscopy
○ Tumor cells are arranged in cribriform pattern
○ Tumor cells have dark, compact nuclei and scant cytoplasm
○ Cribriform spaces are filled with hyaline material

Q6. Write a short note on nasopharyngeal carcinoma.

Ans.
Nasopharyngeal carcinoma
○ Bimodal age group (15–25 years and 60–69 years)
○ **Etiopathogenesis:** EBV infection, diets rich in nitrosamines and smoking
○ EBV detection is done by: PCR or by FISH (which detects EBV encoded RNA, EBER-1 or proteins such as LMP-1 in malignant epithelial cells)

Three patterns
a. Keratinizing squamous cell carcinomas
b. Non-keratinizing squamous cell carcinomas
c. Undifferentiated carcinomas (lymphoepithelioma)

Treatment
○ **Radiotherapy** is the standard modality of treatment
○ **Undifferentiated carcinoma** is most **radiosensitive**
○ **Keratinizing squamous cell carcinoma** is least radiosensitive

Q7. Write a note on paragangliomas.

Ans.
Paragangliomas
○ Arises from the clusters of neuroendocrine cells
○ In adrenal glands, they are termed pheochromocytoma
○ 70% of **extra-adrenal paragangliomas** occur in the **head and neck** region

Paragangliomas *can develop at:*

a. **Paravertebral paraganglia** (e.g. organs of Zuckerkandl)—innervated by sympathetic nervous system and are chromaffin-positive

b. Paraganglia related to the **great vessels** of the **head and neck** (aorticopulmonary chain): For example, **carotid bodies (most common)**; aortic bodies; jugulotympanic ganglia—innervated by the **parasympathetic** nervous system

Carotid body tumor

○ Arises at the **bifurcation of the common carotid artery**

○ Slow-growing and painless masses

○ Age group: 40–50 years

○ Familial cases are associated with MEN-2 syndrome

Morphology

Microscopy

○ **Composed of nests (Zellballen)** of round to oval chief cells, surrounded by delicate vascular septae

○ **Chief cells** stain strongly for **chromogranin, synaptophysin, neuron-specific enolase**

○ Surrounding the chief cells there occurs spindle-shaped stromal cells (sustentacular cells), which are positive for S-100 protein

16

Gastrointestinal Tract

Q1. Write a note on Meckel diverticulum.

Ans.

Meckel diverticulum
- Most common true diverticulum
- Most common site is ileum
- Occurs due to failed involution of the vitelline duct
- Solitary diverticulum extends from the anti-mesenteric side of the bowel

Rule of "2s"
- Occurs in approximately 2% of population
- Present within 2 feet (60 cm) of the ileocecal valve
- Approximately 2 inches (5 cm) long
- Twice as common in males
- Most often symptomatic by age of 2 years

Q2. Write pathology, morphology and clinical features of Hirschsprung's disease.

Ans.

Hirschsprung's disease

Pathogenesis
- Premature arrest of normal migration of neural crest cells from cecum to rectum
- Absence of Meissner submucosal and Auerbach myenteric plexus ("aganglionosis")
- Peristaltic contractions are absent and functional obstruction occurs
- Results in dilation, proximal to the affected segment

Morphology
- Rectum is always affected
- Aganglionic segment is normal or constricted
- Proximal colon (normal): May undergo progressive dilation, resulting in megacolon
- Intraoperative frozen-section analysis is commonly used for diagnosis
- Microscopy: Absence of ganglion cells within the affected segment

Clinical Features
- Failure to pass meconium in postnatal period
- Abdominal distention and bilious vomiting

Q3. Write a note on Barrett esophagus.
Ans.
Barrett esophagus
- Occurs due to complication of chronic gastroesophageal reflux disease
- Characterized by intestinal metaplasia within the esophageal squamous mucosa
- Associated with an increased risk of esophageal adenocarcinoma

Morphology
- **Gross:** Patches of red, velvety mucosa extending upward from the gastroesophageal junction

Microscopy
- Intestinal-type metaplasia is seen
- Intestinal epithelium replaces the squamous esophageal epithelium and has goblet cells
- On H&E: Goblet cells have distinct mucous vacuoles that stain pale blue
- Dysplasia: Both low grade and high grade dysplasia can be seen

Q4. Discuss etiopathogenesis and morphology of *H. pylori* gastritis.
Ans.
- Most common affected site is **antrum**

Pathogenesis
- Presents as antral gastritis with normal or increased acid production
- Increased risk of duodenal ulcer

Virulence of H. pylori is because of its:
- **Flagella:** Which allows the bacteria to be motile in viscous mucus
- **Urease:** Which generates ammonia from endogenous urea and thereby elevates gastric pH
- **Adhesins:** Enhance bacterial adherence to the surface foveolar cells
- **Toxin:** Cytotoxin-associated gene A (CagA) is responsible for disease progression

Morphology
- Within the stomach, *H. pylori* are most often found in the antrum and is concentrated within the superficial mucus overlying epithelial cells in the surface and neck regions
- Can be detected with special stains like Warthin-Starry **silver stain, Giemsa stain, toluidine blue**

Gastric biopsy shows
- Neutrophils within the lamina propria and intraepithelial neutrophils

○ Pit abscesses and increased plasma cells in the superficial lamina propria

○ Increased numbers of sub-epithelial lymphocytes and macrophages

Q5. Differences between benign and malignant ulcers of stomach.

Ans.

Benign gastric ulcer

○ Peptic ulcer is round to oval, sharply punched-out defect

○ Mucosal margin may overhang the ulcer base

○ Gastric rugae reach close to the ulcer margin

Malignant gastric ulcer

○ Ulcers have characteristic heaped-up margins

○ Gastric rugae stop far away from the ulcer margin

Q6. Discuss in detail the etiopathogenesis and morphology of gastric carcinoma.

Ans.

Pathogenesis

Intestinal type gastric cancer is associated with mutations that result in increased signaling via the Wnt pathway and includes:

○ Loss of function mutations in the adenomatous polyposis coli (APC) tumor suppressor gene

○ Gain-of-function mutations in the gene encoding α-catenin

Diffuse gastric cancer is associated with –

○ Familial gastric cancer—loss-of-function mutations in tumor suppressor gene CDH1, which encodes "E-cadherin"

○ Sporadic gastric cancer—E-cadherin mutation

○ Loss of E-cadherin—key step in the development of "diffuse gastric cancer"

Morphology

○ **Sites**—gastric antrum, lesser curvature is more commonly involved than greater curvature

Gastric cancers with intestinal morphology

○ Presents as an ulcerated tumor or an exophytic mass

○ Tumors are composed of glandular structures

○ Tumor cells contain apical mucin vacuoles and mucin may be present in gland lumina

Gastric cancers with diffuse infiltrative growth pattern

○ Tumors produce a desmoplastic reaction that stiffens the gastric wall, leading to leather bottle appearance termed linitis plastica

○ Composed of signet-ring cells, which are discohesive, with large mucin vacuoles

○ Vacuoles expand the cytoplasm and push the nucleus to the periphery creating a signet-ring cell morphology

Q7. Write a note on carcinoid tumor.

Ans.

Carcinoid tumors
○ Referred as well-differentiated neuroendocrine tumors

Sites
○ Most common site is gastrointestinal tract
○ 40% occur in the small intestine (jejunum and ileum)
○ Tracheobronchial tree and lungs are the next most common sites

Morphology
○ **Gross:** Intramural or submucosal masses that create small polypoid lesions
○ Cut surface: Yellow or tan in color

Microscopically
○ Carcinoids are composed of islands, trabeculae, glands, or sheets of uniform cells with scant, pink granular cytoplasm and a round to oval stippled nucleus
○ Rarely, pleomorphism, anaplasia, mitotic activity and necrosis can be seen
○ Immunohistochemical stains are positive for synaptophysin and chromogranin A

Q8. Discuss intestinal morphology of celiac disease

Ans.

Morphology of celiac disease
○ Biopsy sites: Second portion of duodenum or proximal jejunum

Microscopy
○ Villous atrophy
○ Increased numbers of intraepithelial CD8+ T lymphocytes (intraepithelial lymphocytosis)
○ Crypt hyperplasia

Note
○ Absence of gluten-free diet leads to restoration of normal mucosal histology
○ Associations: Blistering skin lesion, dermatitis herpetiformis

Q9. Write morphology of Whipple disease.

Ans.

Whipple disease
○ Causative agent: Gram-positive actinomycete, *Tropheryma whippelii*

Morphology
○ Hallmark is dense accumulation of distended, foamy macrophages in the small intestinal lamina propria
○ Macrophages contain periodic acid—Schiff (PAS)—positive granules that represent lysosomes stuffed with partially digested bacteria

Note
o Similar infiltrate of foamy macrophages is present in intestinal tuberculosis (PAS-positive organisms), however, mycobacteria shows AFB positivity, while *T. whippelii* does not

Q10. Classify inflammatory bowel diseases. Discuss in detail the gross and micro-scopic morphology of Crohn Disease

Ans.

Inflammatory Bowel Disease
o Includes ulcerative colitis and Crohn disease

Crohn disease
Morphology
o Most common sites involved at presentation are the terminal ileum, ileocecal valve, and cecum
o Earliest lesion: Aphthous ulcer, which may progress into elongated, serpentine ulcers oriented along the axis of the bowel
o Skip lesions: Characteristic feature which helps to differentiate from ulcerative colitis
o Strictures are common
o Cobblestone appearance: Diseased tissue is depressed below the level of normal mucosa
o Fissures develop between the mucosal folds and may lead to development of fistulous tracts
o Creeping fat: Mesenteric fat extends around serosal surface

Microscopy
o Crypt abscesses: Neutrophils within a crypt
o Crypt destruction and distortion of mucosal architecture
o Hallmark of Crohn disease—non-caseating micro-granulomas

Q11. Enumerate the differences between Crohn disease and ulcerative colitis.

Ans.

Differentiating features between ulcerative colitis and Crohn disease

Feature	Crohn disease	Ulcerative colitis
Bowel region	Ileum ± colon	Colon only
Distribution	Skip lesions	Diffuse
Stricture	Present	Absent
Wall appearance	Thick	Thin
Inflammation	Transmural	Limited to mucosa
Pseudo polyps	Moderate	Marked
Ulcers	Deep, knife-like	Superficial, broad-based
Lymphoid reaction	Marked	Moderate

Contd.

Contd.

Feature	Crohn disease	Ulcerative colitis
Fibrosis	Marked	Mild to none
Serositis	Marked	Mild to none
Granuloma	Present	Absent
Fistulae/sinuses	Present	Absent
Perianal fistula	Yes (in colonic disease)	No
Fat/vitamin malabsorption	Seen	Not seen
Malignant potential	With colonic involvement	Yes
Toxic megacolon	Not seen	Seen
Recurrence after surgery	Common	No

Q12. Write a note on Peutz-Jeghers syndrome.

Ans.

Peutz-Jeghers syndrome

○ **Autosomal dominant** syndrome
○ Presents with **multiple GI hamartomatous polyps** and **mucocutaneous hyperpigmentation**
○ Associated with **increased risk of cancers** of the colon, pancreas, breast
○ Occurs due to **loss-of-function mutations** in the gene **LKB1/STK11**
○ **Most common site** of **polyps—small intestine**, followed by stomach, colon, bladder and lungs
○ Microscopic hallmark is **arborizing polyp.**

Q13. Write a note on familial adenomatosis polyposis.

Ans.

Familial adenomatous polyposis (FAP)

○ Autosomal dominant disorder, patients develop numerous colorectal adenomas
○ Caused by mutations of the adenomatous polyposis coli, or APC gene
○ 100 polyps are necessary for a diagnosis of classic FAP
○ Colorectal adenocarcinoma develops in 100% of untreated FAP patients, before 30 years of age
○ Extra-intestinal manifestation: Congenital hypertrophy of the retinal pigment epithelium

Q14. Write about gross and microscopic findings in colon carcinoma.

Ans.

Morphology of colon carcinoma

Gross:

○ Carcinomas in the proximal colon (cecum and ascending colon): Polypoidal, exophytic masses that extend along one wall, and rarely causes obstruction

○ Carcinomas in the distal colon: Annular lesions that produce "napkin-ring" constrictions and luminal narrowing

Microscopy
○ Cuboidal to columnar cells in papillary, glandular and trabecular pattern
○ Pleomorphic nuclei, and increased mitotic activity
○ Desmoplastic stromal response
○ Abundant mucin accumulation can be seen within the intestinal wall
○ Signet-ring cells can be seen

17

Liver and Gallbladder

Q1. Write laboratory diagnosis of hepatitis B.

Ans.

Natural course of hepatitis B

- ○ HBsAg appears before the onset of symptoms, and declines to undetectable levels in 12 weeks
- ○ HBeAg, HBV-DNA, and DNA polymerase appear in the serum soon after HBsAg, and all signify active viral replication
- ○ Anti-HBs antibody titers rise as the titers of HBsAg falls
- ○ Anti-HBs may persist for life, and is the basis for current vaccination strategies using noninfectious HBsAg
- ○ Persistence of HBeAg is an important indicator of continued viral replication
- ○ IgM anti-HBc antibody becomes detectable in the serum shortly before the onset of symptoms, which is replaced by IgG anti-HBc over period of months

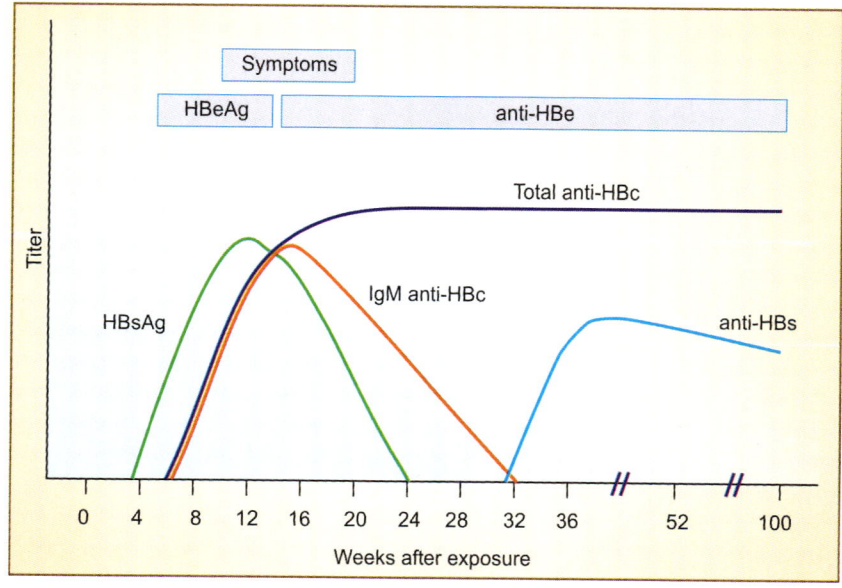

Fig. 17.1: Natural course of hepatitis B infection

Q2. Write a note on CVC liver.

Ans.

Passive congestion and centrilobular necrosis

Right-sided cardiac failure

○ Leads to **passive congestion** of the liver

○ Liver is slightly enlarged, tense, and cyanotic

○ Microscopically: Congestion of centrilobular sinusoids

Left-sided cardiac failure

○ Leads to hepatic hypoperfusion and hypoxia

○ **Centrilobular necrosis**—ischemic coagulative necrosis of hepatocytes in the central region of the lobule (around the central vein)

Centrilobular hemorrhagic necrosis (nutmeg liver)

○ Due to combination of hypo perfusion and retrograde congestion of liver

○ Liver takes on a variegated mottled appearance and resembles like a nutmeg, hence named "nutmeg liver"

Q3. Write a note on cirrhosis of the liver.

Ans.

Cirrhosis

○ A condition marked by diffuse transformation of the entire liver into regenerative parenchymal nodules surrounded by fibrous bands and variable degrees of vascular shunting

How is cirrhosis brought about?

○ Cytokines and chemokines that play a role in cirrhosis of liver include:

  a. Platelet-derived growth factor receptor β (PDGFR-β) results in proliferation and activation of hepatic stellate cells into myofibroblasts

  b. Transforming growth factor β (TGF-β), results in fibrogenetic property of stellate cells

  c. Endothelin-1 (ET-1) results in contraction of myofibroblasts

Microscopic feature of cirrhosis

○ Thick bands of collagen separate rounded cirrhotic nodules

Clinical Features:

○ Jaundice, encephalopathy, coagulopathy

○ Pruritus (in patients with chronic jaundice)

○ Palmar erythema and spider angiomas of the skin: Due to impaired estrogen metabolism and hyperestrogenemia in male patients with chronic liver failure

○ Hypogonadism and gynecomastia in males due to hyperestrogenemia

Q4. Write morphological features of chronic viral hepatitis.
Ans.

Chronic hepatitis
○ Defined as symptomatic, biochemical, or serological evidence of continuing or relapsing hepatic disease for more than 6 months

Microscopy
○ Characteristic feature is mononuclear inflammatory cell infiltrate around the portal tract
○ Interface hepatitis: Inflammatory infiltrate is seen at the interface between the hepatocytes and portal tract
○ Hallmark of progressive chronic liver damage is "scarring"
○ With scarring, there is increased ductular reaction (increase in number of bile ductules)

Chronic hepatitis B
○ Diagnostic hallmark is presence of **"Ground-glass" hepatocytes,** i.e. hepatocytes with endoplasmic reticulum swollen with HBsAg

Chronic hepatitis C
○ Shows lymphoid aggregates or fully formed lymphoid follicles
○ Fatty change of scattered hepatocytes

Q5. Discuss in detail the etiopathogenesis and morphology of alcoholic liver disease.
Ans.

Three forms of alcoholic liver injury
1. Hepatocellular steatosis or fatty change
2. Alcoholic (or steato-) hepatitis
3. Steato-fibrosis, including cirrhosis in the late stages of disease

Pathogenesis
1. Hepatocellular steatosis
   ○ Increased generation of NADPH (lipid biosynthesis) by alcohol dehydrogenase and acetaldehyde dehydrogenase, resulting in impaired lipoprotein synthesis
2. Alcoholic hepatitis
   ○ Alcohol ingestion leads to production of reactive oxygen species (ROS) due to increased cytochrome P-450 metabolism
3. Steatofibrosis
   ○ Alcohol stimulates endothelin release from endothelial cells, resulting in vasoconstriction and contraction of activated stellate cells

Morphology
1. Hepatic Steatosis (Fatty Liver)
   ○ Grossly: Enlarged liver, can weigh as heavy as 4 to 6 kg, appears to be yellow and greasy

○ Microscopy: Lipid droplets accumulate in hepatocytes, begins as small droplets which coalesce into large droplets and push the nucleus aside

2. Alcoholic (steato) hepatitis

○ Hepatocyte swelling and necrosis

○ **Mallory-Denk bodies:** Eosinophilic material in hepatocytes, made up of tangled skins of intermediate filaments such as keratins 8 and 18 in complex with ubiquitin

○ Neutrophilic infiltration of hepatocytes

3. Alcoholic steatofibrosis

○ Occurs due to prominent activation of sinusoidal stellate cells and portal fibroblasts, with resultant fibrosis

○ **Chicken wire fence pattern:** Scarring starts around the sinusoidal hepatocytes and spreads outward, encircling individual or small clusters of hepatocytes

○ End-stage alcoholic liver disease is termed **micro-nodular or Laënnec cirrhosis**

Q6. Discuss the pathogenesis and morphology of hemochromatosis.

Ans.

Hemochromatosis

○ Caused by excessive iron absorption, which gets deposited in liver and pancreas, heart, joints, and endocrine organs

○ Total body iron pool ranges from 2 to 6 gm in normal adults; about 0.5 gm is stored in the liver

○ In most severe forms of hemochromatosis, total iron accumulation may exceed 50 gm, more than one-third of which accumulates in the liver

Leads to

○ Micronodular cirrhosis in all patients

○ Diabetes mellitus

○ Abnormal skin pigmentation

Pathogenesis

○ Disease manifests when more than 20 gm of iron have accumulated

○ Hepcidin secreted by liver is the main regulator of iron absorption

○ Hepcidin lowers plasma iron levels and its deficiency leads to iron overload

○ Adult form of hemochromatosis is caused by mutations of HFE gene, located on the short arm of chromosome 6

Morphology

1. Deposition of hemosiderin occurs in (decreasing order of severity) liver, pancreas, myocardium, pituitary gland, adrenal gland, thyroid and parathyroid glands, joints, and skin

2. Cirrhosis

3. Pancreatic fibrosis

Hematoxylin and eosin stain
- Iron becomes evident as golden-yellow hemosiderin granules in the cytoplasm of periportal hepatocytes

Prussian blue
- Gives blue color to hemosiderin containing hepatocytes

Q7. Write a note on α_1-antitrypsin deficiency.

Ans.

α_1-Antitrypsin deficiency
- Autosomal recessive disorder of hepatocellular accumulation of misfolded proteins due to low levels of circulating α_1-antitrypsin (α_1-AT)
- α_1-AT: Inhibits proteases, neutrophil elastase, cathepsin G, and proteinase 3, which are released from neutrophils at sites of inflammation
- α_1-AT deficiency leads to development of pulmonary emphysema (due to the increased proteases)
- α_1-AT gene is located on chromosome 14 and has different genotypes
- PiMM is the most common genotype, seen in 90% of individuals
- Most common clinically significant mutation is PiZZ
- Homozygotes for PiZZ protein have circulating α_1-AT levels that are only 10% of normal
- Mutant polypeptide α_1-AT-Z, is abnormally folded and polymerized, triggering unfolded protein response, that may lead to apoptosis
- Also there occurs accumulation of misfolded proteins in the liver
- All individuals with PiZZ genotype accumulate α_1-AT-Z in the endoplasmic reticulum of hepatocytes
- Hepatocellular carcinoma develops in 2% to 3% of PiZZ adults
- α_1-AT deficiency is most commonly diagnosed inherited hepatic disorder in infants and children

Morphology
- Presence of round to oval cytoplasmic globular inclusions in the hepatocytes, which are strongly periodic acid–Schiff (PAS) positive and diastase-resistant
- Electron microscopy: Endoplasmic reticulum dilated by aggregates of misfolded proteins

Q8. Write a note on hyperbilirubinemia.

Ans.

Causes of increased bilirubin levels
Unconjugated bilirubin
- Is insoluble in water and exists in complexes with serum albumin
- Hemolytic disease of the newborn (erythroblastosis fetalis) may lead to accumulation of unconjugated bilirubin in the brain, which results in severe neurologic damage, referred to as kernicterus

Causes of unconjugated hyperbilirubinemia

a. *Excess production of bilirubin*
  - Hemolytic anemia, resorption of blood from internal hemorrhage, ineffective erythropoiesis (e.g. pernicious anemia, thalassemia)

b. *Impaired bilirubin conjugation*
  - Physiologic jaundice of the newborn (decreased UGT1A1 activity, decreased excretion)
  - Genetic deficiency of UGT1A1 activity (Crigler-Najjar syndrome types I and II)
  - Gilbert syndrome
  - Diffuse hepatocellular disease (e.g. viral or drug-induced hepatitis, cirrhosis)

Conjugated bilirubin
  - Is water-soluble, nontoxic, and can be excreted in urine
  - Serum bilirubin levels in the normal adult vary between 0.3 and 1.2 mg/dl
  - Jaundice becomes evident when serum bilirubin levels rise above 2 to 2.5 mg/dl

Causes
  - Dubin-Johnson syndrome, rotor syndrome

Q9. Write a note on cholestasis.

Ans.

Cholestasis
  - Caused by impaired bile formation and bile flow with resultant accumulation of bile pigment in the hepatic parenchyma
  - Caused by extra hepatic or intrahepatic obstruction of bile channels

Clinical and lab features
  - Patients may have jaundice, pruritus, skin xanthomas (focal accumulation of cholesterol)
  - Nutritional deficiencies of fat-soluble vitamins A, E, D, or K
  - Characteristic laboratory finding is elevated serum alkaline phosphatase and γ-glutamyl transpeptidase (GGT), enzymes present on the apical (canalicular) membranes of hepatocytes and bile duct epithelial cells

Morphology
  - Accumulation of bile pigment within the hepatocytes is seen
  - Elongated green-brown plugs of bile are visible in dilated bile canaliculi
  - Rupture of canaliculi leads to extravasation of bile, which is phagocytosed by Kupffer cells
  - Droplets of bile pigment accumulate within the hepatocytes, which now appear fine and foamy, called **"feathery degeneration"**

Q10. Write a note on primary biliary cirrhosis.

Ans.

Primary biliary cirrhosis (PBC)

○ **Autoimmune** inflammatory disease with F : M ratio in excess of 6 : 1
○ **Clinical features**—fatigue, pruritus, hepatomegaly, eyelid xanthelasmas, hyper-pigmentation, inflammatory arthropathy and cirrhosis in chronic cases
○ Anti-mitochondrial antibodies are present in **90% to 95% of patients**
○ Elevated levels of **alkaline phosphatase** and **γ-glutamyltransferase** are seen
○ Increased risk of developing **hepatocellular carcinoma**

Extrahepatic manifestations

○ Sjögren syndrome, systemic sclerosis, thyroiditis, rheumatoid arthritis, Raynaud phenomenon, membranous glomerulonephritis, and celiac disease

Q11. Classify hepatocellular adenomas.

Ans.

Hepatocellular adenomas

Risk factors: Oral contraceptives and anabolic steroids

Pathogenesis: 3 subtypes:

a. HNF1-α inactivated hepatocellular adenomas

○ Most commonly found in women
○ No risk of malignant transformation
○ Inactivating mutations of HNF1-α are most commonly seen

b. β-Catenin activated hepatocellular adenomas

○ High risk for malignant transformation
○ Associated with oral contraceptive and anabolic steroid use
○ Activating mutations of β-catenin are seen

c. Inflammatory hepatocellular adenomas

○ Associated with non-alcoholic fatty liver disease (NAFLD)
○ IL-6 mediates JAK-STAT signaling and leads to overexpression of acute phase reactants (C-reactive protein and serum amyloid A)
○ Definitive risk for malignant transformation

Q12. Enumerate the precursor lesions of hepatocellular carcinoma. Discuss etiopathogenesis, and morphology of hepatocellular carcinoma.

Ans.

Precursor lesions of hepatocellular carcinoma

a. Cellular dysplasia (small cell change and **large cell change)**

○ Seen in chronic liver disease

b. Low-grade and **high-grade** dysplastic nodules

○ Seen in **cirrhosis**

Etiopathogenesis
1. **Risk factors**
   - Viral infections (HBV, HCV) and toxic injuries (aflatoxin, alcohol)
   - Hereditary hemochromatosis, α_1-AT deficiency, Wilson disease and metabolic syndrome (associated with obesity, diabetes mellitus, and nonalcoholic fatty liver disease)
2. **Molecular changes seen in hepatocellular carcinoma**
   - β-catenin activation
   - p53 inactivation
   - IL-6/JAK/STAT signal pathway activation

Morphology
Gross
- Can be unifocal or multifocal mass, varying size nodules, or a diffusely infiltrative cancer

Microscopy
- Well-differentiated to highly anaplastic lesions
- Well-differentiated HCCs have cells resembling normal hepatocytes, but with thickened trabecular structures or pseudo-glandular structures

Q13. Write a note on cholangiocarcinoma.

Ans.
Cholangiocarcinoma
- Malignancy of the biliary tree, arising from bile ducts within and outside of the liver

Risk factors
- Infestation by liver flukes (Opisthorchis and Clonorchis species)
- Chronic inflammatory disease of large bile ducts—e.g. primary sclerosing cholangitis
- Hepatitis B and C, and non-alcoholic fatty liver disease

Sites
- Can be intrahepatic or extrahepatic
- Klatskin tumors/extrahepatic tumors (perihilar) are located at the junction of the right and left hepatic ducts

Gross
- Extrahepatic cholangiocarcinoma—appear as firm, gray nodules within the bile duct wall
- Intrahepatic cholangiocarcinoma—occurs in the noncirrhotic liver

Microscopy
- Are typical adenocarcinoma and produce mucin
- Well to moderately differentiated with clearly defined glandular/tubular structures lined by malignant epithelial cells
- Desmoplastic stromal response, lymphovascular and perineural invasion are common

Q14. Write a note on risk factors and pathological effects of gallstones.

Ans.

Two types of gallstones

a. Cholesterol stones: Composed of cholesterol monohydrate
b. Pigment stones: Composed predominantly of bilirubin calcium salts

Risk factors

a. Cholesterol stones
- Female sex hormones: Female gender, oral contraceptives, pregnancy
- Obesity and metabolic syndrome
- Rapid weight reduction
- Gallbladder stasis
- Hyperlipidemia syndromes

b. Pigment stones:
- Chronic hemolytic syndromes
- Biliary infection
- Gastrointestinal disorders: Ileal disease (e.g. Crohn disease), ileal resection or bypass, cystic fibrosis

Pathogenesis

Conditions that lead to formation of **cholesterol gallstones**
- **Supersaturation of bile** with cholesterol
- **Hypomotility** of the gallbladder
- **Hypersecretion of mucus** in gallbladder

Conditions that lead to formation of **pigment stones** (increased **unconjugated bilirubin in bile**):

- **Chronic hemolytic anemia**
- Severe ileal dysfunction
- Infection of the biliary tract with *Escherichia coli*, *Ascaris lumbricoides* or the liver fluke, *Clonorchis sinensis*

18

Pancreas

Q1. Discuss pathogenesis and morphology of acute pancreatitis.

Ans.

Pathogenesis of acute pancreatitis
- Intrapancreatic activation of trypsin, prophospholipase and proelastase

Mechanisms by which activation of these enzymes are brought about

a. *Pancreatic duct obstruction*
   - **Causes:** Gallstones, biliary sludge, pancreatic cancer, choledochoceles, parasites (Ascaris and Clonorchis)
   - Results in activation of lipases, which brings about fat necrosis
   - There occurs resultant interstitial edema, impaired blood flow and ischemia

b. *Primary acinar cell injury*
   - **Causes:** Alcohol, drugs, trauma, ischemia, viruses, hypercalcemia
   - Resulting in release and activation of proenzymes especially trypsin

Genes implicated in hereditary pancreatitis
- Gain-of-function mutations in the trypsinogen gene (also known as PRSS1)
- Loss of function mutations in SPINK1
- Loss of function mutations in the cystic fibrosis transmembrane conductance regulator (CFTR) gene

Morphology of acute pancreatitis

Gross
- Pancreas appears red-black due to hemorrhage with foci of yellow-white, chalky fat necrosis

Microscopy
- Fat necrosis
- Acute inflammation
- Destruction of the pancreatic parenchyma
- Interstitial hemorrhage

Q2. Write a note on chronic pancreatitis.
Ans.

Chronic pancreatitis
- **Definition:** Prolonged inflammation of the pancreas associated with irreversible destruction of exocrine and endocrine parenchyma with accompanying fibrosis

Causes
- Alcohol abuse (most common cause)
- Obstruction of the pancreatic duct by calculi
- Autoimmune injury to the gland
- Hereditary pancreatitis associated with germline mutations in CFTR genes

Pathogenesis
- Chronic pancreatic injury results in stimulation of pancreatic periacinar myofibroblasts which secrete TGF-β and platelet-derived growth factor (PDGF)
- Autoimmune pancreatitis: Associated with the presence of IgG4-secreting plasma cells in the pancreas

Morphology
Microscopy
- Entire pancreatic parenchyma is replaced by fibrotic bands with atrophy of pancreatic islets and ducts
- Interspersed chronic inflammatory cells are seen admixed the sclerotic stroma
- Autoimmune pancreatitis is characterized by increased IgG4 plasma cells

Complications
- Pancreatic pseudocyst
- Chronic malabsorption
- Diabetes mellitus
- Pancreatic cancer (in hereditary pancreatitis)

Q3. Enumerate the pancreatic changes in diabetes mellitus.
Ans.

Morphology of pancreas in type I DM
a. **Insulitis:** Leukocytic infiltrates in the islets
b. Reduction in number and size of the islets

Morphology of pancreas in type II DM
Amyloid deposition within the islets, in and around capillaries and between cells

19

Kidney

Q1. Write characteristic features of nephritic syndrome and nephrotic syndrome.

Ans.

Characteristic features of nephritic syndrome

- Hematuria
- Azotemia
- Proteinuria
- Oliguria
- Edema
- Hypertension

Characteristic features of nephrotic syndrome

- Massive proteinuria: >3.5 gm/day
- Hypoalbuminemia
- Hyperlipidemia
- Lipiduria

Q2. A 12-year-old boy presented with fever, oliguria and high colored urine. He had sore throat three weeks back.

  i. What is your probable diagnosis?

 ii. Describe the etiopathogenesis of the condition.

iii. What are the relevant investigations?

Ans.

Poststreptococcal glomerulonephritis

- Appears 1 to 4 weeks after streptococcal infection of the pharynx or skin
- Most commonly affects the children in between 6 and 10 years of age

Etiology and pathogenesis

- Caused by group A β-hemolytic streptococci, most common subtypes include types 12, 4, and 1

Clinical features

- A young child abruptly develops malaise, fever, nausea, oliguria, and hematuria (smoky or cola-colored urine), 1 to 2 weeks after recovery from sore throat
- Peri-orbital edema, mild to moderate hypertension

Laboratory findings

- Elevated anti-streptococcal antibody titers
- Decline in serum concentration of C3 and other components of the complement cascade

Morphology

- Enlarged, hypercellular glomeruli (diffuse and global)
- Hypercellularity is caused by:
  a. Proliferation of endothelial and mesangial cells
  b. Infiltration by leukocytes

Electron microscopy

- Discrete, amorphous, electron-dense sub-epithelial deposits giving it the appearance of humps (sub-epithelial humps)

Immunofluorescence microscopy

- Granular deposits of IgG and C3, in the mesangium and along the GBM

Q3. Write a note on crescentic glomerulonephritis.

Ans.

Rapidly progressive (crescentic) glomerulonephritis

- Characterized by rapid and progressive loss of renal function
- Most common histologic picture is presence of crescents in most of the glomeruli **(Crescentic glomerulonephritis)**
- Crescents are produced due to proliferation of parietal epithelial cells

Classification

a. *Type I*
  - Goodpasture syndrome

b. *Type II (immune complex)*
  - Post-infectious glomerulonephritis
  - Lupus nephritis
  - Henoch-Schönlein purpura
  - IgA nephropathy

c. *Type III (pauci-immune)*
  - ANCA-associated
  - Granulomatosis with polyangiitis (formerly called Wegener granulomatosis)
  - Microscopic polyangiitis

Microscopy
- Glomeruli shows the presence of crescents

Electron microscopy
- Shows ruptures in the glomerular basement membrane (GBM)

Mechanism of crescent formation
- GBM rupture allows leukocytes, plasma proteins and inflammatory mediators to reach the urinary space, where they trigger formation of crescents

Q4. Write a note on Goodpasture syndrome.

Ans.

Goodpasture syndrome
- Basement membrane is made up of type IV collagen
- Type IV collagen has non-collagenous domains
- If noncollagenous domains of type IV collagen act as an antigen, these individuals are prone to suffer basement membrane damage
- In anti-GBM antibody-induced nephritis, antibodies are formed against the **noncollagenous (NC1) domain of α_3 chain of type IV collagen**
- **Goodpasture disease/syndrome:** These anti-GBM antibodies cross react with other basement membranes, especially in the lung alveoli, resulting in simultaneous lung and kidney injury

Morphology
- Produces a characteristic crescentic glomerulonephritis
- **Electron microscopy** shows rupture in glomerular basement membrane
- **Immunofluorescence:** It shows diffuse linear pattern due to deposition of antibodies along the entire length of **glomerular basement membrane**

Q5. Enumerate the causes of nephrotic syndrome.

Ans.

Causes of nephrotic syndrome

1. **Primary glomerular diseases**
   - Membranous nephropathy, minimal-change disease, focal segmental glomerulosclerosis, membranoproliferative glomerulonephritis and dense deposit disease, IgA nephropathy

2. **Systemic diseases**
   - Systemic lupus erythematosus, diabetes mellitus, amyloidosis, drugs (NSAIDs, penicillamine, "street heroin"), infections (malaria, syphilis, hepatitis B and C, HIV), malignancy (carcinoma, lymphoma)

Q6. Write a note on the pathology of manifestations of nephrotic syndrome.

Ans.

Pathology of manifestations occurring in nephrotic syndrome patients
- Heavy proteinuria depletes serum albumin levels with resultant hypoalbuminemia

○ Decreased intravascular colloid osmotic pressure results in generalized edema

○ **Highly selective proteinuria:** There occurs loss of low-molecular-weight proteins, i.e. albumin, transferrin and anti-thrombin III

○ Increased synthesis of lipoproteins in liver and decreased lipid catabolism results in hyperlipidemia with resultant lipiduria

○ Due to loss of immunoglobulin in urine, patients are prone to develop staphylococcal and pneumococcal infections

○ Loss of endogenous anticoagulants (antithrombin III) in urine, results in thrombotic and thromboembolic complications

Q7. Thirteen-year-old female child had massive edema with puffiness of face with decreased urine output.

a. What is the most probable diagnosis?

b. What can be the most probable renal pathology in this child?

c. Write in detail about minimal change disease.

Ans.

a. Most probable diagnosis is nephrotic syndrome.

b and c.

Minimal change disease

○ Benign disorder, characterized by diffuse effacement of foot processes of visceral epithelial cells

○ Most frequent cause of nephrotic syndrome in children

○ Follows a respiratory infection or routine prophylactic immunization

Morphology

Light microscopy

○ Glomeruli appears normal

Electron microscopy

○ GBM appears normal

○ There occurs uniform and diffuse effacement of foot processes

Immunofluorescence

○ Shows no Ig or complement deposits

Q8. Write a note on Alport's syndrome.

Ans.

Alport's syndrome (X-linked trait)

Patient presents as

○ Hematuria, which can progress to chronic renal failure

○ Nerve deafness

○ Lens dislocation, posterior cataracts, and corneal dystrophy

Pathogenesis
- Mutation of α_5 chain of type IV collagen (COL4A5): X-linked form is seen in 85% of patients
- Mutation of COL4A3 or COL4A4 are seen in AR and AD forms

Electron microscopy
- GBM shows an irregular foci of thickening alternating with attenuation (thinning), and pronounced splitting of lamina densa, producing a distinctive basket weave appearance

Q9. Discuss in detail about diabetic nephropathy.

Ans.

Diabetic nephropathy

Lesions seen in diabetic kidney patients include:

1. Glomerular lesions
2. Renal vascular lesions
3. Pyelonephritis, including necrotizing papillitis

1. **Glomerular lesions include**
   a. *Capillary basement membrane thickening*
      - Widespread thickening of the glomerular capillary basement membrane
      - Thickening of tubular basement membranes
   b. *Diffuse mesangial sclerosis*
      - Diffuse increase in mesangial matrix, depositions of which are PAS positive
   c. *Nodular glomerulosclerosis:*
      - Also known as **Kimmelstiel-Wilson kidney disease** or inter-capillary glomerulosclerosis
      - Glomeruli shows nodular deposits situated at the periphery of the glomerulus, which are PAS-positive
      - Nodular lesions are accompanied by accumulation of hyaline material in the capillary loops ("fibrin caps") or adherent to the Bowman capsules ("capsular drops")
      - Glomerular arteries undergo ischemia, resulting in contraction of the kidney or shrunken kidney

2. **Renal vascular lesions** include atherosclerosis and arteriolosclerosis

3. **Pyelonephritis:** Acute pyelonephritis, i.e. necrotizing papillitis (or papillary necrosis) is much more prevalent in diabetics

Q10. Write a note on diffuse lupus nephritis.

Ans.

Diffuse lupus nephritis (Class IV)
- Most common and severe form of lupus nephritis

- Half or more of the glomeruli are affected
- Involved glomeruli shows proliferation of endothelial, mesangial and epithelial cells
- **Wire loop structures:** Sub-endothelial immune complex deposits leading to circumferential thickening of the capillary wall, on light microscopy

Q11. Write a note on acute tubular necrosis.

Ans.

Acute tubular necrosis

Acute tubular injury/necrosis (ATI/ATN)
- Characterized by necrosis of tubular epithelial cells

Types

a. Ischemic ATI
- **Causes:** Marked hypotension and shock
- **Morphology:** Tubular necrosis is patchy, with straight segments of proximal tubules (PST) and ascending limbs of Henle's loop (HL) being most commonly affected

b. Nephrotoxic ATI
- **Causes:** Drugs (gentamicin), radiographic contrast agents, poisons, including heavy metals (mercury), organic solvents (carbon tetrachloride)
- **Morphology:** Extensive necrosis is present along the proximal convoluted tubule segments (PCT)

Q12. Describe the etiopathogenesis, gross and microscopy of chronic pyelonephritis.

Ans.

Chronic pyelonephritis
- Disorder in which chronic tubulo-interstitial inflammation and scarring involves the calyces and pelvis

Etiopathogenesis
- Acute pyelonephritis is the initiating factor, which occurs following urinary tract infection
- Urinary tract infection is caused by gram-negative bacilli, most commonly by *Escherichia coli*, Proteus, Klebsiella, and Enterobacter

Two forms

1. Reflux nephropathy:
- Vesicoureteral reflux with added infection leads to chronic pyelonephritic scarring

2. Chronic obstructive pyelonephritis:
- Obstruction predisposes the kidney to infection

Morphology

Gross
- Kidneys are irregularly scarred

- Asymmetrical involvement of bilateral kidneys (**Note:** Diffuse and symmetrical scarring of both the kidneys is seen in chronic glomerulonephritis)
- Coarse, discrete, corticomedullary scars with overlying dilated, blunted or deformed calyces, and flattening of the papillae
- Scars are most commonly seen in the upper and lower poles

Microscopy

- Tubules may be atrophic or hypertrophied
- **Thyroidization of tubules:** Dilated tubules filled with casts resembling thyroid colloid
- Chronic interstitial inflammation and fibrosis in the cortex and medulla

Q13. Write a note on xanthogranulomatous pyelonephritis.

Ans.

Xanthogranulomatous pyelonephritis

- Associated with **proteus** infections
- **Gross:** Lesions may produce large, yellowish orange nodules that may be grossly confused with renal cell carcinoma
- **Microscopy:** Characterized by accumulation of foamy macrophages, plasma cells, lymphocytes, polymorphonuclear leukocytes and occasional giant cells

Q14. Discuss in detail about benign nephrosclerosis.

Ans.

Benign nephrosclerosis

- Associated with sclerosis of renal arterioles and small arteries
- Strongly associated with hypertension
- Affected vessels have thickened walls and narrowed lumens, resulting in focal parenchymal ischemia

Pathogenesis

Arterial lesions occur due to:

- Medial and intimal thickening, due to hemodynamic changes, aging, genetic defects
- Hyalinization of arteriolar walls, due to extravasation of plasma proteins through injured endothelium

Morphology

Gross

- Cortical surfaces have fine, even granularity that resembles grain leather
- Loss of mass is due to cortical scarring and shrinking

Microscopy

Hyaline arteriolosclerosis

- Thickening and hyalinization of the arterial walls with resultant narrowing of the lumens of arterioles and small arteries
- Vascular narrowing, leads to patchy ischemic atrophy of the renal parenchyma
- Finely granular surface appears microscopically as sub-capsular scars

Q15. Discuss in detail about malignant nephrosclerosis.

Ans.

Malignant nephrosclerosis:

○ Renal vascular disorder associated with malignant or accelerated hypertension

Pathogenesis

○ Characteristic lesion in malignant nephrosclerosis is vascular injury

Clinical features

○ Characterized by systolic pressures greater than 200 mm Hg and diastolic pressures greater than 120 mm Hg

Morphology

a. Gross

○ Small, pinpoint petechial hemorrhages on the cortical surface, gives the kidney a peculiar "flea-bitten" appearance

b. Microscopy

Two histologic alterations characterize blood vessels in malignant hypertension:

a. Fibrinoid necrosis of arterioles: Vessel wall shows a smudgy eosinophilic appearance due to fibrin deposition

b. Hyperplastic arteriolitis (onion-skin lesion): Intimal thickening due to proliferation of elongated, concentrically arranged smooth muscle cells of intima

Q16. Write a note on polycystic kidney disease.

Ans.

Autosomal dominant (adult) polycystic kidney disease

○ Hereditary disorder characterized by multiple expanding cysts of both the kidneys

○ Cysts destroy renal parenchyma and cause renal failure

Genetics and pathogenesis

1. PKD1 gene:

○ Located on chromosome 16p and encodes polycystin-1

○ PKD1 gene mutation accounts for 85% of cases

2. PKD2 gene:

○ Located on chromosome 4q and encodes polycystin-2

○ Polycystin-2 is expressed in all segments of renal tubules and in many extra-renal tissues

Morphology

Gross

○ Kidneys are **bilaterally** enlarged

○ **External surface**—composed of multiple cysts, varying up to 3 to 4 cm in diameter, with no intervening parenchyma

○ Cysts may be filled with clear, serous fluid or with turbid, red to brown, sometimes hemorrhagic fluid

Extra-renal congenital anomalies seen in patients with polycystic kidney disease:

○ Polycystic liver disease

○ Cysts may occur in spleen, pancreas, and lungs

○ Intracranial berry aneurysms

○ Mitral valve prolapse

Q17. Write a note on Henoch–Schönlein purpura.

Ans.

Henoch–Schönlein purpura

○ Age group affected is 3–8 years

○ Patients have a history of atopy

○ The disease starts after an onset of acute respiratory infection

○ Patient presents as purpuric skin lesions, abdominal pain, intestinal bleeding, and arthralgias along with renal abnormalities

○ Purpuric skin lesions occurs on extensor surfaces of arms, legs and buttocks

○ Abdominal manifestations include pain, vomiting, and intestinal bleeding

○ Renal manifestations include gross or microscopic hematuria and can present as nephritic syndrome, nephrotic syndrome or rarely as crescentic glomerulonephritis

○ Patients have IgA deposits in their mesangium (the resultant picture resembles IgA nephropathy)

Q18. Enumerate different types of renal stones.

Ans.

Four main types of calculi:

a. Calcium stones, composed of calcium oxalate or calcium oxalate mixed with calcium phosphate

b. Triple stones or struvite stones, composed of magnesium ammonium phosphate (forms the largest stones, so-called stag horn calculi)

c. Uric acid stones

d. Cystine stones

Q19. Classify renal cell carcinoma. Enumerate its risk factors. Discuss in detail the morphology of clear cell carcinoma.

Ans.

Classification of renal cell carcinoma

○ Clear cell carcinoma

○ Papillary carcinoma

○ Chromophobe carcinoma

○ Chromosome Xp11 translocation carcinoma

○ Collecting duct carcinoma

○ Medullary carcinoma

Risk factors for renal cell carcinoma

○ Smoking, obesity (in women), hypertension, unopposed estrogen therapy, exposure to asbestos, petroleum products and heavy metals
○ Increased risk in patients with end stage renal disease, chronic kidney disease, acquired cystic disease and tuberous sclerosis

Morphology of clear cell carcinomas

○ Arise from proximal tubular epithelium

Gross

○ Solitary unilateral lesions
○ **Cut surface** appears bright yellow
○ Yellow color is due to prominent lipid accumulation in tumor cells
○ Areas of hemorrhage and necrosis can be seen
○ Margins are sharply defined and are confined within the renal capsule

Microscopy

○ Growth pattern varies from solid to trabecular (cordlike) or tubular (resembling tubules)
○ Tumor cells have rounded or polygonal shape and abundant clear or granular cytoplasm, which contains glycogen and lipids
○ Tumors have delicate branching vasculature
○ Most tumors are well-differentiated, but tumors can show nuclear atypia with bizarre nuclei and giant cells
○ Tumors can invade the renal vein and can extend up to IVC

Q20. Discuss molecular genetics of renal cell carcinoma. Add a note on paraneoplastic syndromes associated with renal cell carcinoma.

Ans.

Molecular genetics of renal cell carcinoma

○ **Sporadic and hereditary clear cell carcinomas:** Chromosome 3 deletion, loss of VHL, mutational inactivation of VHL, hypermethylation of VHL
○ **Sporadic papillary renal cell carcinoma:** Trisomy 7 and 17; loss of Y and mutated, activated MET
○ **Hereditary papillary renal cell carcinomas:** Trisomy 7 and mutated, activated MET
○ **Xp11 translocation carcinoma:** Translocations of the TFE3 gene located at Xp11.2

Paraneoplastic syndromes associated with renal cell carcinoma

○ Polycythemia, hypercalcemia, hypertension, Cushing syndrome, eosinophilia, leukemoid reactions and amyloidosis, feminization or masculinization

20

Lower Urinary Tract and Male Genital Tract

Q1. Write a note on grading of urothelial tumors (seen in urinary bladder).

Ans.

WHO/International Society of Urological Pathology (ISUP) grading of urothelial tumors

○ Urothelial papilloma
○ Urothelial neoplasm of low malignant potential
○ Papillary urothelial carcinoma, low grade
○ Papillary urothelial carcinoma, high grade
○ Carcinoma *in situ*
○ Invasive urothelial cancer

a. **Urothelial papillomas**
   ○ Small superficial exophytic structures attached to the bladder mucosa with a stalk
   ○ Papillae have a central core of loose fibrovascular tissue covered by epithelium, which resembles to normal urothelium histologically

b. **Papillary urothelial neoplasms of low malignant potential (PUNLMP)**
   ○ These tumors are larger than papillomas
   ○ Papillae with a thicker urothelial layer in comparison to papilloma

c. **Low-grade papillary urothelial carcinomas, non-invasive**
   ○ Urothelial cells have orderly architectural and cytological appearance
   ○ Tumor cells are cohesive and show mild nuclear atypia with a few cells showing hyperchromatic nuclei and infrequent mitotic figures

d. **High-grade papillary urothelial cancers, non-invasive**
   ○ Tumor cells are dyscohesive with large hyperchromatic nuclei
   ○ Atypical mitotic figures are frequent
   ○ These tumors can show invasion into the muscular layer

e. **Carcinoma** *in situ*
- Can present as reddening, granularity and thickening of the bladder mucosa
- Tumor cells lack cohesiveness and can be easily shed in urine
- *Microscopy*: It shows presence of cytologically malignant tumor cells within a flat urothelium

f. **Invasive urothelial cancer:**
- Highly atypical pleomorphic tumor cells with invasion into the deeper muscular layers
- Extent of the invasion into the muscularis mucosae is of prognostic significance

Q2. Write a note on etiopathogenesis of transitional cell carcinoma of bladder.

Ans.

Factors implicated in causation of bladder cancer/ transitional cell carcinoma
- Cigarette smoking
- Industrial exposure to arylamines
- Schistosoma hematobium infection
- Long-term use of analgesics
- Heavy long-term exposure to cyclophosphamide
- Pelvic irradiation for other cancers
- Genetic alterations:
  - Gain of function mutations in FGFR3
  - Loss of function mutations in TP53 and RB tumor suppressor genes
  - Activating mutations in HRAS oncogene
  - Monosomy or deletions of chromosome 9p and 9q

Q3. Write a short note on condyloma acuminata (warts) affecting male genital tract.

Ans.

Condyloma acuminatum
- **Causative agent** (sexually transmitted disease): Human papillomavirus (HPV) type 6 and 11
- **Site and gross features:** Most commonly affect coronal sulcus and inner surface of the prepuce, where they present as single or multiple, sessile or pedunculated, red papillary excrescences

Microscopy
- Lesion is composed of branching, villous, papillary connective tissue stroma, covered by the epithelium with hyperkeratosis and acanthosis (thickening of the underlying epidermis)
- Surface epithelium shows characteristic viral cytopathic change/ koilocytic atypia
- **Koilocytic atypia:** Manifests as nuclear enlargement, hyperchromasia and a cytoplasmic perinuclear halo

Q4. Write a short note on Bowen disease.

Ans.

Bowen disease

- Affects males more than 35 years of age
- **Site**: Involves the skin of the shaft of the penis and the scrotum

Gross: Solitary, thickened, gray-white, opaque plaque

Microscopy

- Epidermis appears hyperplastic
- Cells in the stratum spinosum shows full thickness epithelial dysplasia with large hyperchromatic nuclei and lack orderly maturation with numerous mitosis
- Basement membrane is intact
- Can transform into infiltrating squamous cell carcinoma

Note

- Bowen disease of glans is termed erythroplasia of Queyrat

Q5. Write a short note on cryptorchidism.

Ans.

- **Definition:** Complete or partial failure of intra-abdominal testes to descend into the scrotal sac
- Undescended testis is at a greater risk of developing testicular cancer than is the descended testes

Two phases of testicular descent

a. Trans-abdominal phase
- Testis comes to lie within the lower abdomen or brim of the pelvis
- Controlled by a hormone called müllerian-inhibiting substance

b. Inguinoscrotal phase
- Testes descend through the inguinal canal into the scrotal sac
- Occurs due to release of calcitonin gene related peptide from the genitofemoral nerve
- Most common site of arrest is in the inguinal canal

Morphology
- Unilateral in most cases, bilateral in 25% of patients

Microscopy
- Altered morphological changes in testes appears as early as 2 years of age
- Characterized by maturation arrest of germ cells
- Tubules show only Sertoli cells
- Marked hyalinization and thickening of the basement membrane of the tubules
- Leydig cells appear prominent

Treatment

○ **Orchiopexy** (placement in the scrotal sac) should be done preferably before 2 years of age
○ Orchiopexy does not guarantee fertility and development of cancer in testes
○ Cancer may also develop in the contralateral, normally descended testis

Q6. Classify germ cell tumors. Discuss gross and microscopic picture of seminoma testis.

Ans.

Germ cell tumors

a. Seminomatous tumors
  ○ Seminoma
  ○ Spermatocytic seminoma
b. Non-seminomatous tumors
  ○ Embryonal carcinoma
  ○ Yolk sac (endodermal sinus) tumor
  ○ Choriocarcinoma
c. Teratoma
d. Sex cord-stromal tumors
  ○ Leydig cell tumor
  ○ Sertoli cell tumor

Seminoma

○ Most common type of germ cell tumor
○ Seen most commonly in third decade
○ Ovarian counterpart of seminoma is dysgerminoma
○ Contains iso-chromosome 12p
○ Expresses OCT3/4 and NANOG
○ 25% of these tumors have activating KIT mutations

Morphology

Gross

○ Produce bulky masses
○ Cut surface: Appears homogeneous, gray white, lobulated
○ Hemorrhage or necrosis is not seen

Microscopy

○ Tumor is composed of sheets of uniform tumor cells
○ Tumor cells are divided into poorly demarcated lobules by delicate fibrous septa
○ The fibrous septae contain lymphocytic infiltrate
○ Tumor cells are large, round to polyhedral, has distinct cell membrane; clear or watery-appearing cytoplasm, large, central nucleus with one or two prominent nucleoli

Q7. Write a short note on spermatocytic seminoma.

Ans.

Spermatocytic seminoma

o Slow growing tumor

o Affects individuals older than age 65 years

o Excellent prognosis

o Gross: Soft, gelatinous appearance

Microscopy

Three cell populations

a. Medium-sized cells (most numerous) containing a round nucleus and eosinophilic cytoplasm with a characteristic spireme chromatin (which resembles that of spermatocytes in meiotic phase)

b. Smaller cells resembling small lymphocytes

c. Scattered giant cells, either uninucleate or multinucleate

Q8. Write a note on pathogenesis and morphology of benign prostatic hypertrophy.

Ans.

Benign prostatic hyperplasia (BPH)

Etiopathogenesis

o Hyperplasia occurs due to impaired cell death rather than increased epithelial cell proliferation

o Androgens required for development of BPH, increases cellular proliferation and inhibits cell death

o Dihydrotestosterone (DHT) is the major androgen in the prostate

o DHT is formed in the prostate from testosterone by the action of an enzyme called type 2 5α-reductase

o This enzyme is located in stromal cells

o Hence, stromal cells are responsible for androgen-dependent prostatic growth

o DHT binds to the nuclear androgen receptors (AR) present in both stromal and epithelial prostate cells

o DHT is more potent than testosterone because it has a higher affinity for AR

o Binding of DHT to AR stimulates the transcription of androgen-dependent genes, which includes several growth factors and their receptors

o DHT-induced growth factors act by increasing the proliferation of stromal cells and decreasing the epithelial cell death

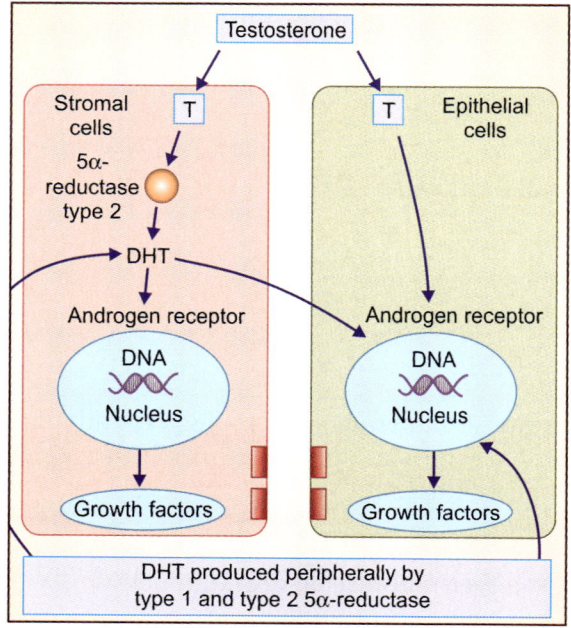

Fig. 20.1: Pathogenesis of benign prostatic hyperplasia

Q 9. Write a short note on prostatic intraepithelial neoplasm.

Ans.

Prostatic intraepithelial neoplasm (PIN)

○ Also called prostatic carcinoma *in situ*

○ Involves prostatic ducts and acini

○ Divided into three grades: PIN I, II, III

○ Categories: PIN I and PIN II—low grade, PIN III—high grade

○ Morphological differentiation between low grade and high grade is based on: Cell crowding and stratification; nuclear enlargement, pleomorphism, and chromatin pattern; and appearance of nucleoli

○ High-grade PIN has an association with prostatic adenocarcinoma

21

Female Genital Tract

Q1. Write a short note on embryonal rhabdomyosarcoma of vagina.

Ans.

Embryonal rhabdomyosarcoma

○ Also called sarcoma botryoides
○ Age group: Infants and children younger than 5 years of age
○ Tumor grows as polypoidal, rounded, bulky masses
○ Appears as grape-like clusters (hence the designation botryoides, or grape-like)

Microscopy

○ Composed of tumor cells containing undifferentiated round or spindle cells in a myxoid stroma
○ Cytoplasm of tumor cells can show striations (indicative of muscle differentiation)
○ **Characteristic feature** is the presence of 'cambium layer' which is a distinctive sub-epithelial dense zone and separates tumor cells from the squamous epithelium

Q 2. Write a short note on cervical intraepithelial neoplasia (CIN).

Ans.

Cervical intraepithelial neoplasia (squamous intraepithelial lesions):

Classification systems for squamous cervical precursor lesions:

Dysplasia/carcinoma in situ	Cervical intraepithelial neoplasia (CIN)	Squamous intraepithelial lesion (SIL), current classification
Mild dysplasia	CIN I	Low-grade SIL (LSIL)
Moderate dysplasia	CIN II	High-grade SIL (HSIL)
Severe dysplasia	CIN III	High-grade SIL (HSIL)
Carcinoma *in situ*	CIN III	High-grade SIL (HSIL)

Morphology

Squamous intraepithelial lesion (SIL)

○ Characterized by nuclear enlargement, hyperchromasia, coarse chromatin and variation in nuclear size and shape

Grading of SIL

○ LSIL (CIN I) is characterized by koilocytic atypia (nuclear alterations with a perinuclear halo) and involves lower one-third of the epithelial thickness

○ HSIL (CIN II) is characterized by progressive atypia and expansion of immature basal cells above the lower third of the epithelial thickness

○ HSIL (CIN III) is characterized by diffuse atypia, loss of maturation and expansion of the immature basal cells to the epithelial surface, i.e. full thickness dysplasia

Q3. A 40-year-female presents with post-coital bleeding and foul smelling discharge per vagina. She also complaints of loss of 15% body weight in the past 2 months, accompanied by loss of appetite.

a. What is your diagnosis?

b. What etiopathogenesis of this condition?

c. What are the morphological features?

d. Write staging of the disease, which patient is suffering from?

Ans.

a. Diagnosis is squamous cell carcinoma of cervix

b. Pathogenesis of squamous cell carcinoma cervix:

○ High-risk HPVs (most commonly HPV-16 and 18) are the most important factors in the development of cervical cancer

○ HPVs infect immature basal cells of the squamous epithelium, in areas of epithelial breaks, or immature metaplastic squamous cells present at the squamocolumnar junction

○ HPVs replicate in mature squamous cells

○ HPV is carcinogenic due to its viral proteins E6 and E7

HPV E6 protein:

○ Leads to degradation of p53, which results in uncontrolled stimulation of cyclin/cyclin-dependent kinases and thus increased cell cycle proliferation

○ Stimulates the expression of TERT, the catalytic subunit of telomerase and inhibits cell death

HPV E7 protein:

○ Binds to the RB protein and displaces the E2F transcription factors that are normally sequestered by RB, promoting the progression of cell cycle

○ Inactivates the CDK inhibitors p21 and p27, which result in uncontrolled stimulation of cyclin/cyclin-dependent kinases and thus increased cell cycle proliferation

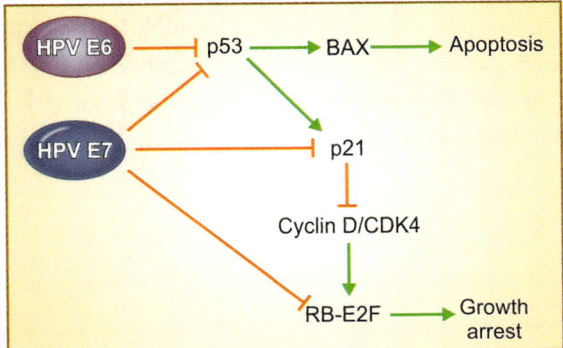

Fig. 21.1: Role of HPV E6 and E7 in cervical carcinoma

c. Morphology

Gross
- Can present either as fungating (exophytic) or infiltrative masses

Microscopy
- Squamous cell carcinoma is composed of nests of malignant squamous epithelium (keratinizing or non-keratinizing) which invades the underlying cervical stroma

Staging of cervical cancer

Stage 0: Carcinoma *in situ* (CIN III, HSIL)

Stage I: Carcinoma confined to the cervix
- Ia: Preclinical carcinoma (diagnosed only by microscopy)
- Ia1: Stromal invasion, no deeper than 3 mm and no wider than 7 mm (so called microinvasive carcinoma)
- Ia2: Maximum depth of invasion of stroma deeper than 3 mm; horizontal invasion not more than 7 mm
- Ib: Histologically invasive carcinoma confined to the cervix and greater than stage Ia2

Stage II: Carcinoma extends beyond the cervix but not to the pelvic wall. Carcinoma involves the vagina but not the lower third

Stage III: Carcinoma has extended to the pelvic wall. On rectal examination there is no cancer-free space between the tumor and the pelvic wall. The tumor involves the lower third of the vagina

Stage IV: Carcinoma has extended beyond the true pelvis or has involved the mucosa of the bladder or rectum. This stage also includes the cancers with metastatic dissemination

Q4. Write a short note on endometriosis.

Ans.

Endometriosis
- **Definition:** Presence of "ectopic" endometrial tissue at a site outside the uterus

○ Abnormal tissue includes both endometrial glands and stroma
○ **Sites:** Ovaries, uterine ligaments, rectovaginal septum, cul-de-sac
○ **Clinical features:** Infertility, dysmenorrhea (painful menstruation), pelvic pain, dyspareunia (pain while intercourse)

Pathogenesis

1. *Regurgitation theory*
   ○ Endometrial tissue implants at ectopic sites via retrograde flow of menstrual endometrium

2. *Benign metastases theory*
   ○ Endometrial tissue from the uterus can "spread" to the distant sites (e.g. bone, lung, and brain) via blood vessels and lymphatic channels

3. *Extra-uterine stem/progenitor cell theory*
   ○ Stem/progenitor cells from the bone marrow differentiate into endometrial tissue

Morphology

○ Presents as red-blue to yellow-brown nodules on mucosal and/or serosal surfaces
○ Ovaries (chocolate cysts or endometriomas) are distorted by large cystic masses (3 to 5 cm in diameter) which are filled with brown fluid resulting from previous hemorrhage
○ Histological diagnosis is made when both endometrial glands and stroma are present in the biopsy studied

Q5. Write a short note on adenomyosis.

Ans.

Adenomyosis

○ **Definition:** Presence of endometrial tissue within the uterine wall (myometrium)
○ **Microscopy:** Irregular nests of endometrial stroma, with or without glands, are present within the myometrium, separated from the basalis layer by at least 2 to 3 mm
○ **Clinical features:** Menometrorrhagia (irregular and heavy menses), colicky dysmenorrhea, dyspareunia, and pelvic pain

Q6. Classify endometrial carcinomas. Write a note about malignant mixed müllerian tumor.

Ans.

Carcinoma of endometrium

Type I (endometrial) carcinoma

○ Most common type
○ Well-differentiated type
○ Mimic proliferative endometrial glands
○ Referred to as endometrioid carcinoma

- Arises in the setting of endometrial hyperplasia
- Associated with: Unopposed estrogen, obesity, hypertension, diabetes

Type II (serous) carcinoma

- Includes serous carcinoma (most common), clear cell carcinoma and malignant mixed müllerian tumor
- Occurs in older women
- Arises in the setting of endometrial atrophy
- Poorly differentiated (grade 3) tumors

Malignant mixed müllerian tumors (MMMTs)

- Also called carcinosarcomas
- Endometrial adenocarcinoma with a malignant mesenchymal component

Morphology

- **Gross:** Tumors are bulky and polypoidal, which protrude through the cervical os
- **Microscopy:** Tumors usually consist of adenocarcinoma (endometrioid, serous or clear cell) mixed with the malignant mesenchymal (sarcomatous) elements
- Sarcomatous components may include striated muscle, cartilage, adipose tissue, and bone
- Metastases contain only epithelial components

Q7. Write a short note on Leiomyoma uteri.

Ans.

Leiomyoma

- Uterine leiomyoma (fibroid) is the most common tumor in women
- Benign smooth muscle neoplasm which may occur singly, or often multiple

Chromosomal abnormality

- Rearrangements of chromosomes 12q14 and 6p involving the HMGIC and HMGIY genes respectively are seen
- Mutations in MED12 gene are common

Morphology

Gross

- Sharply circumscribed, discrete, round, firm, gray-white tumors varying in size from small nodules to massive tumors
- **Fibroids can be:** Intramural (within the myometrium), sub-mucosal (just beneath the endometrium) or sub-serosal (beneath the serosa)

Cut surface

- Characteristic whorled pattern of smooth muscle bundles

Microscopy

- Leiomyomas are composed of bundles of smooth muscle cells
- Individual muscle cells have characteristic oval nucleus and long, slender bipolar cytoplasmic processes

○ Variants:
  a. Atypical or bizarre tumors with nuclear atypia and giant cells
  b. Cellular leiomyomas

Clinical features

○ Abnormal bleeding, increased urinary frequency (due to compression of the bladder), sudden pain from infarction of a large or pedunculated tumor, and impaired fertility

○ Myomas in pregnant women increases the frequency of spontaneous abortion, fetal mal-presentation, uterine inertia (failure to contract with sufficient force), and postpartum hemorrhage

Q8. Classify ovarian neoplasms. Discuss in detail the molecular pathogenesis and morphology of serous tumors.

Ans.

WHO classification of ovarian neoplasms

1. Surface epithelial-stromal tumors
  a. *Serous tumors*
    ○ Benign, borderline, malignant
  b. ***Mucinous tumors**, endocervical-like and intestinal type*
    ○ Benign, borderline, malignant
  c. *Endometrioid tumors*
    ○ Benign, borderline, malignant (endometrioid adenocarcinoma)
  d. *Clear cell tumors*
    ○ Benign, borderline, malignant
  e. *Transitional cell tumors*
    ○ Benign Brenner tumor, Brenner tumor of borderline malignancy, malignant Brenner tumor
  f. *Epithelial-stromal*
    ○ Adenosarcoma, malignant mixed müllerian tumor

2. Sex cord-stromal tumors
  ○ Granulosa cell tumors, fibromas, fibrothecomas, thecomas, Sertoli-Leydig cell tumors, steroid (lipid) cell tumors

3. Germ cell tumors
  ○ Teratoma—immature, mature {solid, cystic (dermoid cyst)}, monodermal (e.g. struma ovarii, carcinoid)
  ○ Dysgerminoma
  ○ Yolk sac tumor (endodermal sinus tumor)
  ○ Mixed germ cell tumors

4. Metastatic cancer from non-ovarian primary
  ○ Colonic, appendiceal, gastric, pancreaticobiliary, breast

Etiopathogenesis of serous epithelial tumors
- **Age group:** 20–45 years (benign and borderline), old age (carcinomas)
- **Risk factors for serous carcinomas:** Nulliparity, family history, and heritable mutations
- Oral contraceptives and tubal ligation reduces the risk
- BRCA-1 and BRCA-2 increase susceptibility to ovarian cancer and predisposes to high grade serous carcinomas

Associations of serous carcinomas
- **Serous tubal intraepithelial carcinoma (STIC):** Occurs in association with high-grade serous ovarian cancers
- Serous ovarian carcinomas arise from cortical inclusion cysts

Morphology of serous epithelial tumors
a. **Benign tumors**
  - **Gross:** Ovary shows a smooth glistening cyst wall with small papillary projections
  - **Microscopy:** Tumor shows stromal papillae, lined by columnar epithelium
b. **Borderline tumors**
  - **Gross:** Ovary is replaced by a cystic cavity, lined by delicate papillary tumor growths
  - **Microscopy:** Tumor cells arranged in papillae with increased architectural complexity and epithelial cell stratification with mild nuclear atypia
c. **Malignant tumors**
  - **Gross:** Ovary shows larger areas of solid or papillary tumor mass
  - **Microscopy:** Tumor cell invasion into the adjacent stroma is seen

Q9. Discuss morphological features of mucinous tumors of ovary.

Ans.
Mucinous tumors
- Comprises 2–25% of all ovarian neoplasms
- Most commonly benign and borderline tumors

Pathogenesis
- Mutation of the **KRAS proto-oncogene** is commonly seen

Morphology
- 5% of primary mucinous cystadenomas and mucinous carcinomas are bilateral

Gross
- Appears as multi-loculated cystic masses, with the cysts being filled with gelatinous fluid (can weigh>25 kg)

Microscopy
Classified into 2 types:
a. **Intestinal type:** Characterized by a papillary architecture lined by tall non-ciliated cells with basal nuclei and abundant intracellular mucin

b. Endocervical type: Characterized by epithelial lining with a 'picket-fence' appearance (columnar cells lining the cysts)

Borderline mucinous tumors

○ Atypical epithelium is less than four cells in thickness (>4 cell thickness is carcinoma)

Malignant mucinous tumor

○ Characterized by cell atypia, increased cell thickness, greater complexity of the glands and papillae (budding, bridging, appearance of solid foci), with areas of stromal invasion

Q10. Write a note on pseudomyxoma peritonei.

Ans.

Pseudomyxoma peritonei

○ Mucinous tumors involving the ovary

○ Characterized by extensive deposits of intra-abdominal mucin

○ Previously, pseudomyxoma peritonei was thought to be due to spread from mucinous ovarian neoplasm

○ But recently it has been shown that it occurs due to metastasis in ovary from appendix (most commonly)

Note

○ Mucinous ovarian tumors are mostly unilateral

○ Hence, in bilateral ovarian tumors, metastatic ovarian carcinoma has to be ruled out

Q11. Write a note on Brenner tumor.

Ans.

Transitional cell tumor (Brenner tumor)

○ Contains neoplastic epithelial cells resembling the urothelium and are mostly benign

Gross

○ Solid or cystic

○ 90% are unilateral

○ Can range in diameter from 1 cm to 20 to 30 cm

Microscopy

○ Ovarian stroma contains sharply demarcated nests of epithelial cells resembling the epithelium of urinary tract

Q12. Discuss in detail the morphology of dermoid cyst of ovary. Mention the components of struma ovarii.

Ans.

Teratomas

a. Mature (benign) teratomas

○ Are cystic, so called dermoid cysts (lined by skin-like structures)
○ Seen in reproductive age group women

Morphology
○ Bilateral in 10–15% of cases

Gross
○ Unilocular cysts containing hair and sebaceous material
○ In the wall, teeth-like structures and areas of calcification are commonly seen

Microscopy
○ Derivatives of all three germ cell layers are seen
○ Cyst wall is composed of stratified squamous epithelium with underlying sebaceous glands, hairshafts, and other skin adnexal structures
○ Cartilage, bone, thyroid, and neural tissue are commonly seen
○ Malignant transformation, most commonly to **squamous cell carcinoma** or thyroid carcinoma, melanoma can occur

Struma Ovarii
○ Monodermal or specialized teratomas
○ Ovarian stroma is composed of mature thyroid tissue

Q13. Discuss dysgerminoma of ovary.

Ans.
Dysgerminoma
○ Malignant tumor
○ Ovarian counterpart of testicular seminoma
○ Occurs in the second and third decades
○ Elevated HCG levels can be seen (due to syncytiotrophoblastic giant cells)
○ Express OCT-3, OCT4, and NANOG
○ Activating mutations in KIT gene are seen

Morphology
○ Unilateral tumors
○ **Cut surface:** Multinodular, solid yellow-white, soft and **fleshy**

Microscopy
○ Tumor cells grow in sheets or cords separated by scant fibrous stroma, which is infiltrated by mature lymphocytes
○ Tumor cells are large vesicular, with clear cytoplasm, well-defined cell boundaries, and a centrally placed regular nuclei

Q14. Write a note on endodermal sinus tumor.

Ans.
Yolk sac tumor (endodermal sinus tumor)
○ Neoplasm of children and young adults
○ Tumor cells elaborate **α-fetoprotein**

Gross
- Tumors can measure up to 15 cm in diameter
- Outer surface is smooth and glistening
- Cut surface: Variegated (heterogeneous), composed of cystic areas admixed with areas of hemorrhage and necrosis

Microscopy
- A glomerulus-like structure composed of a central blood vessel enveloped by tumor cells within a space that is also lined by tumor cells (**Schiller-Duval body**)
- Intracellular and extracellular hyaline droplets are present

Q15. Write important features of sex cord stromal tumors.
Ans.
Sex cord stromal tumors
- Tumors are derived from the ovarian stroma (which is derived from sex cords of embryonic gonads)
- Gonadal mesenchyme produces Sertoli cells and Leydig cells in males and granulosa cells and theca cells in females
- As Leydig cells secrete androgens, their corresponding tumors produce masculinizing symptoms
- As granulosa and theca cells secrete estrogens, their corresponding tumors produce feminizing symptoms

Clinical features of Sertoli-Leydig cell tumors
- **Defeminization:** Atrophy of the breasts, amenorrhea, sterility, and loss of hair
- Musculinization: Virilization (hirsutism) with male distribution of hair, hypertrophy of the clitoris, and voice change

Q16. Discuss in detail about granulosa cell tumor of ovary
Ans.
Granulosa cell tumors
- Resembles granulosa cells of developing ovarian follicle
- **Two types**: Adult and juvenile granulosa cell tumors
- Most commonly seen in **postmenopausal women**

Morphology
Gross
- Unilateral, large, solid, cystic encapsulated mass
- Cut surface: Appears yellow due to intracellular lipids

Microscopy
- Tumor cells grow in anastomosing cords, sheets, or nests
- Tumor cells are small, cuboidal to polygonal
- **Call-Exner bodies:** Small, distinctive, gland-like structures filled with an acidophilic material

Clinical features
○ Elaborate large amounts of estrogen
○ Are potentially malignant
○ Juvenile granulosa cell tumors in pre-pubertal girls may lead to precocious sexual development
○ In adults, they may be associated with proliferative breast disease, endometrial hyperplasia, and endometrial carcinoma
○ Elevated tissue and serum levels of inhibin (a product of granulosa cells) are seen
○ **FOXL2** positivity is seen in adult granulosa cell tumor, but it is negative in juvenile granulosa cell tumor

Q17. Mention briefly about Krukenberg tumor.

Ans.

Krukenberg tumor
○ Metastatic gastric carcinoma involving bilateral ovaries
○ Microscopy: Metastases composed of mucin-producing, signet ring cancer cells

Q18. Write a note on hydatidiform mole.
Ans.
Hydatidiform mole
○ Associated with an increased risk of persistent trophoblastic disease (invasive mole) or choriocarcinoma
○ Two types—complete and partial
a. **Complete mole**
   ○ Results from fertilization of an ovum that has lost its female chromosomes
   ○ Genetic material is paternally derived
   ○ **Androgenesis:** 90% have 46, XX karyotype due to the duplication of the genetic material of one sperm
   ○ 10% result from the fertilization of an empty egg by two sperms; these may have 46, XX or 46, XY karyotype
   ○ Fetal parts are not identified as embryo dies early
   ○ Increased risk for choriocarcinoma and persistent or invasive mole
   Gross
   ○ Delicate friable mass of cystic, grape-like structures, which are villi showing hydropic degeneration
   Microscopy
   ○ Chorionic villi are enlarged, scalloped in shape with central cavitation (cisterns)
   ○ Circumferential trophoblastic proliferation around the individual villi
b. **Partial mole**
   ○ Occurs as a result from fertilization of an egg with two sperms
   ○ In these moles, the karyotype is triploid (e.g. 69, XXY)

○ Fetal tissues are typically present

○ Partial moles have an increased risk of persistent molar disease

○ **Not associated with increased risk of choriocarcinoma**

Microscopy

○ Fraction of villi is enlarged and edematous

○ Focal trophoblastic hyperplasia

○ Villi have an irregular, scalloped outline and contain vessels with fetal (nucleated) red blood cells

Q19. Describe in detail about choriocarcinoma.

Ans.

Choriocarcinoma

○ Malignant neoplasm of trophoblastic cells derived from previously normal or abnormal pregnancy (extra-uterine ectopic)

○ Rapidly invasive and metastasizes widely

○ 50% arise in complete hydatidiform moles, 25% in previous abortions, 22% follow normal pregnancies, and remaining in ectopic pregnancies

Morphology

Gross: Soft, fleshy, yellow-white tumor with large areas of necrosis and extensive hemorrhage

Microscopy

○ Tumor is composed of clusters of cytotrophoblasts and syncytiotrophoblasts

○ Hemorrhage and necrosis are usually present

○ Villi are characteristically absent

○ Tumor invades the underlying myometrium, penetrates blood vessels, and can extends out onto the uterine serosa and into the adjacent structures

Clinical Features

○ Manifests as irregular vaginal spotting of a bloody, brown fluid

○ Hematogenous spread is common

○ Widespread metastases is characteristic

○ Most common sites of metastasis include lungs, vagina, followed by brain, liver, bone and kidney

○ HCG levels are elevated and the levels are above those seen in hydatidiform moles

○ **Treatment:** Evacuation of the contents of the uterus followed by chemotherapy

Q20. Write a note on sites of ectopic gestation.

Ans.

Ectopic gestation

○ Refers to implantation of the fetus at a site other than the normal intrauterine location

○ Most common site is extrauterine fallopian tube (90% of cases)
○ Other sites include ovary, abdominal cavity, and the intrauterine portion of the fallopian tube (cornual pregnancy)
○ Causes of ectopic gestation: Pelvic inflammatory disease, peritubal scarring and adhesions, intrauterine contraceptive device usage

Note: Rupture of tubal pregnancy is medical emergency

22

Breast

Q1. Write a note on fibrocystic disease of breast.

Ans.

Fibrocystic disease

Three principal morphologic changes seen are:

1. **Cystic change**
   - ○ **Gross:** Cysts contain turbid, semi-translucent fluid of brown or blue color, and are called blue dome cysts
   - ○ **Microscopy:** Cysts are lined by apocrine cells with round nuclei and abundant granular cytoplasm
   - ○ Mammography reveals calcifications
   - ○ Mass disappears after FNAC
2. **Fibrosis**
   - ○ Cysts may rupture, resulting in leakage of contents into adjacent stroma
   - ○ Leakage of contents brings about a chronic inflammatory reaction and concomitant scarring, resulting in palpable nodularity
3. **Adenosis**
   - ○ Increase in number of acini per lobule

Q2. Write a note on gynecomastia.

Ans.

Gynecomastia

- ○ It is defined as enlargement of the male breast
- ○ **Cause:** Increased estrogen levels as seen in cirrhosis of liver
- ○ **Microscopically:** Increase in dense collagenous connective tissue associated with ductal epithelial hyperplasia

Q3. Mention the risk factors of carcinoma breast.

Ans.

Risk factors

a. **Germline mutations**
b. **First-degree relatives with breast cancer:** Risk is not increased if the only affected relative is postmenopausal mother

c. **Race/ethnicity**

d. **Age: 70–80 years**

e. **Age at menarche:** Young age at menarche and late menopause

f. **Age at first livebirth:** Pregnancy before 20 years of age reduces the risk than nulliparous women or mothers more than 35 years of age

g. **Benign breast disease:** Atypical hyperplasia or proliferative changes in breast increase the risk of invasive carcinoma

h. **Estrogen exposure**
   - Menopausal hormone therapy increases the risk
   - Oral contraceptives do not appear to increase the risk
   - Oophorectomy, anti-estrogenic drugs (tamoxifen) or aromatase inhibitors reduce the risk

i. **Breast density:** High breast density increases the risk

j. **Radiation exposure:** Risk is greatest with exposure at young ages

k. **Carcinoma of the contralateral breast or endometrium:** Due to excess estrogen

l. **Diet:** Excess alcohol increases the risk

m. **Obesity**
   - <40 years—decreased risk, due to anovulatory cycles
   - Postmenopausal females: Increased risk

n. **Breastfeeding:** Lactation suppresses ovulation and trigger the terminal differentiation of luminal cells, thus reducing the risk

Q4. Discuss etiopathogenesis of familial breast cancers.

Ans.

Familial breast cancers
   - BRCA1, BRCA2, TP53, and CHEK2—tumor suppressor genes involved in familial breast cancers and have a role in DNA repair

a. *BRCA-1 mutation*
   - Located on chromosome 17q21
   - Increased risk of female breast, ovarian, male breast cancer (lower than BRCA2), prostate, pancreas and fallopian tube cancers
   - Breast carcinomas are poorly differentiated and have medullary features
   - Tumors are triple negative (basal-like), i.e. ER-negative and HER2-negative

b. *BRCA-2 mutation*
   - Located on chromosome 13q12–13
   - Increased risk for female breast cancer, ovarian cancer, male breast cancer (more than BRCA1), prostate, pancreas, stomach, melanoma, gallbladder, bile duct, pharynx cancers
   - Poorly differentiated cancers, but are more often ER-positive than BRCA1 cancers

c. *Germline mutations in TP53 (Li-Fraumeni syndrome)*
- Most commonly mutated gene in the sporadic breast cancers
- Most frequent in triple negative cancers
- Associated cancers include: Sarcoma, leukemia, brain tumors, adrenocortical carcinoma

d. *CHEK-2 mutations*
- Increase the risk for breast cancer after radiation exposure
- 70–80% are ER-positive
- Associated with prostate, thyroid, kidney and colon cancers

Q5. Mention the types of breast cancers.

Ans.

- More than 95% of breast malignancies are adenocarcinoma

a. **Carcinoma** *in situ*
- Neoplastic proliferation of epithelial cells that are confined to the ducts and lobules by the basement membrane
- Includes ductal carcinoma *in situ* and lobular carcinoma *in situ*

b. **Invasive carcinoma ("infiltrating" carcinoma)**
- Has penetrated through the basement membrane and grows within stroma
- Includes infiltrating ductal carcinoma (most common variant)

Q6. Write a note on Paget disease of the nipple.

Ans.

Paget disease of the nipple
- Rare manifestation of breast cancer
- Presents as a unilateral erythematous eruption with pruritis
- Lesion may be mistaken for eczema
- From the DCIS lesion, these cells spread to the skin of the nipple via the lactiferous sinuses without crossing the basement membrane and are called Paget cells
- Tumor cells disrupt the normal epithelial barrier, and allow extracellular fluid to seep out onto the nipple surface
- 50 to 60% of women with Paget's disease, have an underlying invasive carcinoma, presenting as a palpable mass
- These invasive carcinoma are poorly differentiated (ER-negative, HER2 over-expression)

Q7. Discuss in detail molecular subtyping of infiltrating breast cancers with examples.

Ans.

Molecular subtypes of invasive breast cancers

1. **ER-positive, HER2-negative** (i.e. **"luminal"**)

○ Most common form of invasive breast cancer

○ Includes low proliferation and high proliferation cancers (associated with BRCA-2 gene mutations)

2. **HER2-positive (20% of cancers)**

○ Second most common molecular subtype of invasive breast cancer

○ Can show germline TP53 mutations

3. **ER-negative, HER2-negative tumors ("basal-like" triple negative carcinoma; 15% of cancers)**

○ Associated with BRCA-1 gene mutations

Examples

a. **ER-positive, HER2-negative (low proliferation) cancers**

○ Well to moderately differentiated mucinous, papillary, cribriform, and lobular carcinomas

b. **ER-positive, HER2-negative (high proliferation) cancers**

○ Includes poorly differentiated lobular carcinoma

c. **HER2-positive cancers**

○ Poorly differentiated cancers, e.g. apocrine cancers and micropapillary cancers

d. **ER-negative, HER2-negative cancers**

○ Poorly differentiated cancers, e.g. squamous cell, spindle cell, medullary, adenoid cystic, metaplastic carcinomas

Q8. Discuss the grading of invasive breast cancers.

Ans.

○ Microscopic grading of the breast carcinoma is done by **Nottingham modification of the Bloom-Richardson system**

Scoring is done on the basis of

a. Tubule formation

b. Nuclear pleomorphism

c. Mitotic rate

○ Carcinomas are graded into grade I (well differentiated), grade II (moderately differentiated), and grade III (poorly differentiated) types

○ **Grade I carcinomas (well-differentiated carcinoma)** grow in a tubular pattern with small round nuclei and low proliferative rate

○ **Grade II carcinomas (moderately differentiated carcinoma)** show some tubule formation, but solid clusters or single infiltrating cells are also present, with greater degree of nuclear pleomorphism and mitotic figures

○ **Grade III carcinomas (poorly differentiated carcinoma)** show tumor cells present in solid sheets of cells with enlarged irregular nuclei, high mitotic rate and frequent areas of tumor necrosis

Parameter	Score 1	Score 2	Score 3
Tubule formation	>75%	10–75%	<10%
Nuclear pleomorphism	Minimal variation	Moderate variation	Marked variation
Mitotic count	0–9	10–19	>20

If total score is 3–5: Grade I; Score 6–7: Grade II; Score 8–9: Grade III

Q9. Write a note on comedo carcinoma breast.

Ans.

Comedo carcinoma

Gross

○ Presents as a mass in the duct, through which the necrotic material can extrude out, hence termed comedone

Microscopy

○ Involved duct is enlarged in size and are lined by atypical pleomorphic tumor epithelial cells, with increased mitotic activity

○ Duct lumen is filled with necrotic material, which can also show areas of coarse calcification

○ Surrounding these ducts, myoepithelial cells are also visible

Note

○ Areas of definite stromal invasion and intra-ductal spread to the nipple (Paget's disease) should always be looked for

Q10. Discuss in detail the prognostic indicators of breast carcinomas.

Ans.

Prognostic indicators

a. **Invasive carcinoma versus carcinoma *in situ* (CIS):** CIS has excellent prognosis

b. **Distant metastases:** If present, indicates poor prognosis

c. **Lymph node metastases**

○ Axillary lymph node status is the most important prognostic factor for invasive carcinomas in the absence of distant metastases

○ Lymphatic vessels in most breast carcinomas drain first to sentinel nodes

d. **Tumor size**

○ Risk of axillary lymph node metastases increases with the size of the primary tumor

e. **Locally advanced disease**

○ Carcinomas invading into skin or skeletal muscle are difficult to treat surgically

f. **Inflammatory carcinoma**

○ Edematous skin is adhered to the breast by Cooper's ligament and mimics the surface of an orange peel, an appearance referred to as peau d'orange

- o Occurs due to dermal lymphatic being filled with metastatic carcinoma
- o Poor prognosis

g. **Lymphovascular invasion:** Poor prognostic factor

h. **Molecular subtype**
- o ER and HER-2 expression and proliferation has different prognostic implications
- o ER and PR positive cancers respond well to hormonal therapy and less to chemotherapy
- o ER or PR negative cancers respond poorly to hormonal therapy but responds well to chemotherapy
- o **HER2 overexpression** is associated with poorer survival

i. **Special histologic types**
- o Tubular, mucinous, lobular, papillary, adenoid cystic carcinomas have better prognosis than NOS type
- o Metaplastic cancers and micro-papillary cancers have worse prognosis

j. **Histologic grade**
- o Nuclear grade, tubule formation, and mitotic rate classify invasive carcinomas into three groups

k. **Proliferative rate**
- o Carcinomas with high proliferation rates (Ki-67 positivity) have poorer prognosis, but responds better to chemotherapy

Q11. Write a note on fibroadenoma.

Ans.

Fibroadenoma
- o Most common benign tumor of the female breast
- o Presents as a palpable mass, can be multiple and bilateral

Morphology

Gross
- o Size: Less than 1 cm to tumors that replace entire breast
- o Tumors are well circumscribed, grayish white nodules, which on cut surface shows slit-like spaces

Microscopy
- o Intra-lobular stroma is delicate and myxoid
- o **Pericanicular pattern:** Epithelium is surrounded by stroma
- o **Intra-canicular pattern:** Epithelial is compressed and distorted by stroma

Q12. Write a note on phyllodes tumor.

Ans.

Phyllodes tumor/cystosarcoma phyllodes
- o Arises from intra-lobular stroma

○ Age group: Sixth decade

○ Associated with gain in the chromosome 1q

○ HOXB13 over-expression is associated with higher tumor grade

Gross

○ Small to massive tumors

Microscopy

○ Composed of nodules of proliferating stroma covered by epithelium

○ Distinguished from fibroadenoma on the basis of higher cellularity, higher mitotic rate, nuclear pleomorphism, stromal overgrowth, and infiltrative borders

Note

○ High grade phyllodes are difficult to differentiate from malignant sarcomas

23

Endocrine System

Q1. Write a note on pituitary adenoma.

Ans.

Pituitary adenoma
- Most common cause of hyperpituitarism
- Can range in size from less than 1 cm (microadenomas) to more than 1 cm (macroadenoma)

Genetic abnormalities
- **G-protein mutations** are the most common alterations
- Cyclin D1 overexpression and RB gene mutation are also seen
- HRAS mutations can be seen

Morphology

Gross
- Soft and well-circumscribed
- Small adenomas—confined to the sella turcica
- Large lesions—extend superiorly into the suprasellar region, compresses the optic chiasm and cranial nerves

Microscopy
- Uniform, polygonal cells arranged in sheets or cords, without supporting connective tissue or reticulin

Note
- In non-neoplastic anterior pituitary parenchyma, cellular monomorphism and absence of significant reticulin network is not seen as seen in pituitary adenomas

Q2. Write a note on craniopharyngiomas

Ans.

Craniopharyngiomas
- Arise from the vestigial remnants of Rathke pouch

○ Bimodal age distribution: First peak at 5 to 15 years of age and second peak at 65 years or older

○ Associated with Wnt signaling pathway abnormalities

Morphology

○ 3 to 4 cm in diameter, cystic and multiloculated

○ Adamantinomatous craniopharyngioma (seen in children) and papillary craniopharyngioma (seen in adults)

Two types

a. Adamantinomatous craniopharyngioma

○ Nests or cords of stratified squamous epithelium, with palisading of squamous epithelium at the periphery

○ Compact, lamellar keratin formation ("wet keratin") is a diagnostic feature

○ Dystrophic calcification is a frequent finding

○ Cyst formation is common and contains cholesterol-rich, thick brownish yellow fluid compared to "machine oil"

b. Papillary craniopharyngioma

○ Solid sheets and papillae lined by well-differentiated squamous epithelium

○ Lacks keratin, calcification, and cysts

○ Peripheral palisading of squamous epithelium is absent

Q3. Define cretinism. Enumerate the causes of hypothyroidism.

Ans.

Cretinism

○ Hypothyroidism that develops in infancy or early childhood

Causes of hypothyroidism

a. Primary

○ Genetic defects in thyroid development (PAX8, TSH receptor mutations)

○ Post-ablative, surgery, radioiodine therapy, or external irradiation

○ Hashimoto thyroiditis, iodine deficiency

○ Drugs (lithium, iodides, p-amino salicylic acid)

○ Dyshormonogenetic goiter (inborn errors of thyroid metabolism)

b. Secondary (central)

○ Pituitary failure

○ Hypothalamic failure

Q4. What is thyroid storm?

Ans.

Thyroid storm

○ It is a medical emergency

○ Characterized by abrupt onset of severe hyperthyroidism in patients with underlying Graves' disease

○ Results from an acute elevation of catecholamines, due to infection, surgery, cessation of antithyroid medication, or stress

○ Patients are febrile and there is tachycardia out of proportion to fever

Q5. Discuss pathogenesis and morphology of Hashimoto thyroiditis.

Ans.

○ Most common cause of hypothyroidism in areas where iodine levels are sufficient

○ Age group: 45 to 65 years

○ F: M:: 10 : 1 to 20 : 1

Pathogenesis

○ Destruction of thyroid follicular epithelial cells by CD8+ T cells or CD4+ T-helper cells

○ Presence of circulating auto-antibodies against thyroglobulin and thyroid peroxidase

○ Polymorphisms in cytotoxic T lymphocyte-associated antigen-4 (CTLA4) and protein tyrosine phosphatase-22 (PTPN22)

Morphology

Gross

○ Diffuse enlargement of thyroid gland

○ Cut surface—nodular, pale, yellow-tan, firm

Microscopy

○ Extensive infiltration of thyroid parenchyma by mononuclear inflammatory infiltrate containing small lymphocytes, plasma cells, and well-developed germinal centers

○ Thyroid follicular epithelial cells show abundant eosinophilic, granular cytoplasm, termed Hürthle cells

Q6. Write a short note on Graves' disease.

Ans.

Graves' disease

○ Most common cause of endogenous hyperthyroidism

○ Age group: 20-40 years, F:M:: 10:1

Triad of:

a. Hyperthyroidism associated with diffuse enlargement of the gland

b. Infiltrative ophthalmopathy with resultant exophthalmos

c. Localized, infiltrative dermopathy, called pretibial myxedema

Pathogenesis

○ Autoimmune disorder characterized by auto-antibodies against TSH receptor

○ Most common antibody detected is **thyroid stimulating immunoglobulin (TSI)**

○ **TSI** binds to TSH receptor and increases the release of thyroid hormones

○ Polymorphisms in CTLA4, PTPN22 genes and HLA-DR3 allele are noted

Morphology

Gross
- Diffuse symmetric enlargement of the thyroid gland
- **Cut surface:** Soft, **meaty** appearance resembling muscle

Microscopy
- Follicles are lined by tall, columnar epithelium
- Epithelial cells project into the lumens of the follicles and actively reabsorb the colloid, resulting in the scalloped appearance of the edges of the colloid
- Interstitium consists of lymphocytes and plasma cells

Q7. Write a note on colloid goiter.

Ans.

Colloid goiter
- Also called diffuse non-toxic (simple) goiter
- Two forms: Endemic and sporadic
1. **Endemic goiter**
   - Prevalent in more than 10% of population in a given region
   - Occurs due to dietary iodine deficiency or due to goitrogens (Cruciferae family, i.e. cabbage, cauliflower, Brussels sprouts, turnips, and cassava)
2. **Sporadic goiter**
   - Female preponderance
   - Peak incidence at puberty or young adulthood

Morphology

Gross
- Enlarged lobes of thyroid glands, whose cut surface is brown, glassy, and translucent

Microscopy
a. **Hyperplastic phase**
   - Thyroid gland is diffusely and symmetrically enlarged
   - Follicles are lined by crowded columnar cells
b. **Colloid involution**
   - If dietary iodine is increased, follicular epithelial cells involutes (epithelial lining is cuboidal or flattened) to form an enlarged, colloid-rich gland **(colloid goiter)**

Q8. Classify neoplasms of thyroid. Write in detail about papillary carcinoma of thyroid.

Ans.

Major neoplasms of thyroid gland
- Papillary carcinoma
- Follicular carcinoma
- Anaplastic (undifferentiated) carcinoma
- Medullary carcinoma

Papillary carcinoma of thyroid
o Most common form of thyroid cancer
o **Age group:** 25–50 years, associated with previous exposure to ionizing radiation

Pathogenesis
o **RET gene** on chromosome 10 shows fusion with **PTC gene** on chromosome 17, resulting in **RET/PTC fusion gene proteins** with increased tyrosine kinase activity
o Gain-of-function mutation in the **BRAF gene**
o BRAF mutations correlate with **metastatic disease** and **extra thyroidal extension**

Morphology
Gross
o Solitary or multifocal, well-circumscribed and encapsulated
o Cut surface: Shows papillary structures

Microscopy
o Branching papillae with fibrovascular stalk covered by single to multiple layers of cuboidal epithelial cells, which can show features of anaplasia
o Nuclei of papillary carcinoma cells appear optically clear and are termed **ground glass** or **Orphan Annie eye nuclei**
o **Intranuclear inclusions** ("pseudo-inclusions")—due to invaginations of the cytoplasm
o **Intranuclear grooves** due to deep infolding of nuclear membranes
o **Psammoma bodies:** Concentrically calcified structures, within the cores of papillae can be seen

Variants of papillary carcinoma of thyroid: Follicular variant, tall cell columnar variant, diffuse sclerosing variant, papillary microcarcinomas

Q9. Write a note on thyroglossal duct cyst.

Ans.
Thyroglossal duct cyst
o Characterized by cystic dilation of thyroglossal duct
o Location: Midline of neck, in the region of the hyoid bone

Microscopy
o Cyst wall is lined by pseudo stratified ciliated or squamous epithelium
o Mucus glands and thyroid follicles are commonly seen in the subjacent stroma

Q10. Write briefly on types of hyperparathyroidism.

Ans.
Three types
a. **Symptomatic primary hyperparathyroidism**
   o Bone disease and pain **(painful bones)**
   o Nephrolithiasis **(renal stones)**
   o Constipation, nausea, peptic ulcers, pancreatitis, gallstones **(abdominal groans)**
   o Depression, lethargy, and seizures **(psychic moans)**
   o **Neuromuscular symptoms:** Weakness and fatigue

b. **Secondary hyperparathyroidism**
- Increase in serum PTH levels, seen in patients with chronic hypocalcemia
- Hypocalcemia leads to compensatory overactivity of the parathyroid glands
- Cause: Chronic renal failure

c. **Tertiary hyperparathyroidism**
- Parathyroid activity may become autonomous and excessive, with resultant hypercalcemia
- **Cause:** Secondary hyperparathyroidism leads to adenoma formation, resulting in autonomous PTH secretion

Q11. Mention skeletal changes in hyperparathyroidism.

Ans.

a. **Osteoporosis**
- Bones involved: Phalanges, vertebrae and proximal femur
- Affects cortical bone more severely than medullary bone
- **Dissecting osteitis:** Osteoclasts dissect centrally along the length of the trabeculae, creating the appearance of railroad tracks

b. **Brown tumors**
- Bone loss predisposes to micro fractures and secondary hemorrhages, resulting in influx of macrophages followed by reparative fibrous tissue

c. **Osteitis fibrosa cystica (von Recklinghausen disease of bone):**
- Hallmark of severe hyperparathyroidism
- Combination of increased osteoclastic activity, peritrabecular fibrosis, and cystic brown tumors

Q 12. Write WHO criteria for diagnosing diabetes mellitus.

Ans.

WHO diagnostic criteria for diabetes include
- Fasting plasma glucose ≥126 mg/dl
- Random plasma glucose ≥200 mg/dl
- 2-hour plasma glucose ≥200 mg/dl during an oral glucose tolerance test (OGTT) with a loading dose of 75 gm
- Glycated hemoglobin (HbA1C) level ≥ 6.5%

Q13. Write a note on actions of insulin.

Ans.

Metabolic actions of insulin

a. *Striated muscle*
- Increased glucose uptake
- Increased glycogen synthesis
- Increased protein synthesis

b. *Liver*
- Decreased gluconeogenesis

- ○ Increased glycogen synthesis
- ○ Increased lipogenesis

c. *Adipose tissue*
- ○ Increased glucose uptake
- ○ Increased lipogenesis
- ○ Decreased lipolysis

Q14. Describe etiopathogenesis of diabetes. What are its complications?

Ans.

Pathogenesis of type 1 diabetes mellitus
- ○ Autoimmune disease resulting in islet cell destruction

a. Genetic susceptibility
- ○ HLA-DR3 or HLA-DR4 haplotype, concurrently with HLA-DQ 8 haplotype, increases the risk
- ○ Variable number of tandem repeats (VNTRs) in insulin gene
- ○ Polymorphisms in CTLA4 and PTPN22 genes

b. Environmental factors
- ○ Viral infection can trigger an immune response, which results in antibody production and thus destruction of islet tissues

Note
- ○ Auto-antibodies against islet antigens are found in majority of patients with type 1 diabetes

Pathogenesis of type 2 diabetes mellitus

a. Genetic factors
- ○ Polymorphisms in genes associated with insulin secretion

b. Environmental factors
- ○ Obesity and sedentary lifestyle leads to insulin resistance

Complications of diabetes
- ○ **Diabetic macrovascular disease:** Resulting in increased risk of myocardial infarction, stroke, and lower extremity ischemia
- ○ **Diabetic microvascular disease:** Resulting in diabetic retinopathy, nephropathy, and neuropathy

Q15. Discuss in detail about the pathogenesis of chronic complications of diabetes.

Ans.

Pathogenesis of chronic complications
- ○ HbA1C provides a measure of glycemic control over the lifespan of a red cell (120 days)
- ○ HbA1C levels should be maintained below 7% in diabetic patients

Mechanisms by which end organ damage is brought

1. Formation of advanced glycation end (AGE) products

○ AGE binds to its receptor (RAGE), which is expressed on endothelium, vascular smooth muscle, and inflammatory cells. Effects of AGE-RAGE complex in vessel walls:

a. Release of TGF β, leading to deposition of excess basement membrane material

b. Release of VEGF, resulting in neovascularisation and is implicated in retinopathy

c. Generation of reactive oxygen species (ROS) in endothelial cells

d. Increased proliferation of vascular smooth muscle cells

2. Activation of protein kinase C

○ Hyperglycemia results in increased production of diacylglycerol (DAG)

○ Increased DAG results in activation of intracellular protein kinase C (PKC), which in turn stimulates the production of VEGF, TGF-β by the vascular endothelium

3. Oxidative stress and disturbances in polyol pathways

○ Glucose is metabolized to sorbitol by aldol reductase and sorbitol is reduced to fructose (a reaction that uses NADPH as cofactor)

○ NADPH is also required by enzyme glutathione reductase in a reaction that regenerates reduced glutathione (GSH)

○ Reduction in GSH, results in increased cellular susceptibility to ROS ("oxidative stress")

○ In hyperglycemia, intracellular NADPH is utilized by aldol reductase

○ Hence, there is reduced GSH regeneration, resulting in oxidative stress

○ Also, sorbitol can show accumulation in the lens, resulting in cataract formation

Q16. Write a note on macrovascular complications seen in diabetes.

Ans.

Macrovascular complications in diabetes

○ Endothelial dysfunction results in accelerated atherosclerosis involving the aorta and large- and medium-sized arteries

○ Results in myocardial infarction (most common cause of death in diabetics), gangrene of the lower extremities

○ **Hyaline arteriolosclerosis:** Amorphous, hyaline thickening of the wall of arterioles, resulting in narrowing of the lumen of the vessel wall

Q17. Write a note on diabetic microangiopathy.

Ans.

Diabetic microangiopathy

○ **Diffuse thickening of basement membrane** is seen in the capillaries of the skin, skeletal muscle, retina, renal glomeruli, medulla and tubules, Bowman capsule, peripheral nerves

○ Resulting in diabetic nephropathy, retinopathy, and neuropathy

Diabetic nephropathy (already discussed in kidney chapter)
o Glomerular lesions; arteriolosclerosis; pyelonephritis

Diabetic ocular complications
o **Hyperglycemia** resulting in formation of cataract, glaucoma, diabetic retinopathy

Diabetic neuropathy
o Peripheral neuropathy, depends on the duration of the diabetes

Q18. Write a note on Zollinger-Ellison syndrome.
Ans.
Zollinger-Ellison syndrome (gastrinomas)

Sites
o **Gastrinoma triangle:** Sites from which they can arise include pancreas, duodenum and peripancreatic soft tissues

Morphology
o More than half of the gastrin-producing tumors are locally invasive or shows metastasis at the time of diagnosis (hepatic metastasis)

Characteristic features
o Marked gastric acid secretion, results in peptic ulceration
o Multiple duodenal and gastric ulcers, which are unresponsive to therapy
o Ulcers can also be seen in unusual locations such as the jejunum

Clinical features
o Similar to symptoms of peptic ulcer disease
o More than 50% patients present with diarrhea

Q19. Write a note on Addison's disease.
Ans.
Addison's disease (primary chronic adrenocortical insufficiency)

Pathogenesis
a. **Autoimmune adrenalitis**
   o Most common cause of primary adrenal insufficiency in developed countries
   o Includes autoimmune polyendocrine syndrome type 1 (APS1) and APS2
b. **Infections**
   o Tuberculosis (most common in India), *Histoplasma capsulatum* and *Coccidioides immitis* and in HIV patients (MAC bacteria, CMV infections)
c. **Metastatic neoplasms**
   o Most common sources include lung and breast carcinomas

Q20. Discuss pheochromocytoma.

Ans.

Pheochromocytoma

○ Neoplasms composed of chromaffin cells, which synthesize catecholamines

Rule of 10s

○ Ten percent of pheochromocytomas are extra-adrenal, called paragangliomas
○ Ten percent of sporadic adrenal pheochromocytomas are bilateral
○ Ten percent of adrenal pheochromocytomas are malignant
○ Ten percent of adrenal pheochromocytomas are not associated with hypertension

Genetics

○ Associated genetic mutations: RET, NF1, VHL, SDHD, SDHC, SDHB (succinate dehydrogenase)

Morphology

Gross

○ Small, circumscribed lesions confined to the adrenal gland to large hemorrhagic masses, which can weigh between 1 gm and 4000 gm (average: 100 gm)
○ **Cut surface:** Appears tan brown to hemorrhagic
○ Incubation of fresh tissue with potassium dichromate solution turns the tumor a **dark brown color**, due to oxidation of stored catecholamines

Microscopy

○ Clusters of polygonal to spindle shaped chromaffin cells, that are surrounded by sustentacular cells, creating small nests or alveoli (zell-ballen)
○ Cells are supplied by rich vascular network
○ Nuclei are round to ovoid, with a stippled "salt and pepper" chromatin
○ **IHC markers:** Chromaffin cells shows chromogranin and synaptophysin positivity, and peripheral sustentacular cells show S-100 positivity

Q21. Write a note on MEN-I and MEN-II syndromes.

Ans.

Multiple endocrine neoplasia, type 1 (MEN-1, or Wermer syndrome)

Etiology

○ **MEN-1 syndrome** is caused by germline mutations in MEN1 tumor suppressor gene, which encodes a protein called menin

Characteristic features

○ Abnormalities of parathyroid, pancreas and pituitary glands

a. Parathyroid

   ○ Primary hyperparathyroidism: Most common manifestation of MEN-1
   ○ Due to parathyroid hyperplasia and adenomas

b. Pancreas
  ○ Endocrine tumors of the pancreas are commonly seen in MEN-1
  ○ Pancreatic polypeptide is the most commonly secreted product
c. Pituitary
  ○ Prolactinoma is the most frequent anterior pituitary tumor

Note
○ In individuals with MEN-1, duodenum is the most common site of gastrinomas

Multiple endocrine neoplasia, type 2
Genetics
○ MEN-2A and MEN-2B are caused by germline gain-of-function mutations in RET proto-oncogene
○ Three distinct syndromes: MEN-2A, MEN-2B, and familial medullary thyroid cancer

MEN-2A, or Sipple syndrome
○ Characterized by pheochromocytoma, medullary carcinoma of thyroid, and parathyroid hyperplasia

MEN-2B
○ Characterized by medullary carcinoma of thyroid, pheochromocytoma, ganglioneuromas (involving the skin, oral mucosa, eyes, respiratory tract and gastrointestinal tract) and marfanoid habitus

24

Skin

Q1. Discuss in detail about the pathogenesis and morphology of malignant melanoma.

Ans.

Pathogenesis

○ Autosomal dominant transmission

○ **Predisposing environmental factor**: Ultraviolet radiation (UVR) resulting in DNA damage

Molecular genetics

a. Mutations that disrupt cell cycle control genes

○ Loss of p16/INK4a expression and CDK4 mutations

b. Increase in RAS and PI3K/ AKT signaling and BRAF mutations

c. Mutations that activate telomerase

○ TERT mutation leads to reactivation of telomerase activity

Morphology

○ Melanomas appear as shades of black, brown, red, dark blue, and gray lesions with irregular and often notched up borders

○ **Radial growth phase:** Horizontal spread of melanoma within the epidermis and superficial dermis

○ **Vertical growth phase:** Tumor cells invade downward into the deeper dermal layers as an expansile mass

○ Tumor cells are larger than normal melanocytes and have large nuclei with irregular contours

○ Nuclear chromatin is clumped at the periphery of the nuclear membranes, with prominent eosinophilic nucleoli

Q2. Discuss the prognostic factors and clinical features of malignant melanoma.

Ans.

I. Prognostic factors

a. Tumor depth (Breslow thickness)

○ Distance from the superficial epidermal granular cell layer to the deepest intradermal tumor cells

○ Probability of metastasis correlates with the depth of invasion

Level of invasion is assessed by Clarke's five level:

Level I: Intra-epidermal (*in situ*) melanocytes

Level II: Extension of melanoma cells in the papillary dermis

Level III: Melanoma cells filling the papillary dermis and stopping at the interphase between the papillary and reticular dermis

Level IV: Melanocytes invading the reticular dermis

Level V: Invades the subcutaneous fat

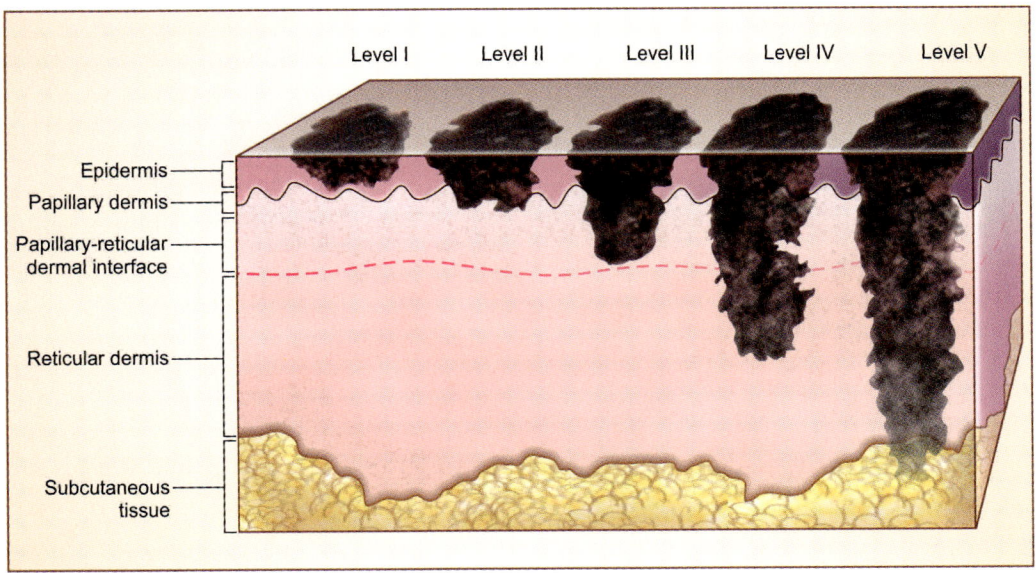

Fig. 24.1: Clarke levels

b. Mitosis: Less mitotic index is a favorable prognostic factor

c. Tumor regression (due to the host immune response): Absence of regression indicates good prognosis

d. Ulceration of the overlying skin: Lack of ulceration is a favorable prognostic factor

e. Presence and number of tumor infiltrating lymphocytes—a brisk tumor infiltrating lymphocyte response indicates favorable prognosis

f. **Sentinal lymph node biopsy:** Microscopic involvement of a sentinel node by small number of melanoma cells (micrometastases) confers a worse prognosis

II. Clinical features (warning signs, i.e. ABCDE of melanoma)

○ **A**symmetry
○ Irregular **b**orders
○ Variegated **c**olor
○ Increasing **d**iameter
○ **E**volution or change over time

Q3. Discuss the pathogenesis and microscopic features of basal cell carcinoma.

Ans.

Basal cell carcinoma

○ Slow growing, locally aggressive cutaneous tumor, that rarely metastasize

Pathogenesis

○ Associated with **nevoid basal cell carcinoma syndrome**: Basal cell carcinoma, medulloblastomas, ovarian fibromas, jaw cysts
○ NBCCS and basal cell carcinoma patients have loss of function mutations of tumor suppressor gene PTCH

Morphology

Gross

○ Presents as pearly papules with prominent dilated sub-epidermal blood vessels (telangiectasias)
○ **Rodent ulcers:** Advanced lesions may ulcerate, and extensive local invasion of the bone or facial sinuses may occur

Microscopy

○ Tumor cells resemble basal cell layer of the epidermis
  a. **Multifocal growth pattern:** Tumor cells proliferate superficially in the epidermis
  b. **Nodular growth pattern:**
○ Basophilic tumor cells grow deep into the dermis and are arranged in cords and islands
○ Tumor cells have a hyperchromatic nuclei and are embedded in a mucinous matrix, surrounded by fibroblasts and lymphocytes
○ Peripheral palisading of tumor cells is seen
○ Retraction clefts which occur when the stroma retracts away from tumor cells

Q4. Write a note on morphology of psoriasis.

Ans.

Morphology of psoriasis

○ **Site:** Elbows, knees, scalp, lumbosacral areas, intergluteal cleft, and glans penis
○ **Early lesions:** Dominated by the presence of small pustules and erythema

○ **Chronic lesions:** Erythematous and covered by a characteristic silver-white scale
○ **Nail changes:** Yellow-brown discoloration, with pitting, dimpling, and onycholysis

Microscopy
○ Acanthosis (marked epidermal thickening), with elongation of rete ridges (appears like test tubes in a rack)
○ Thinning or absent stratum granulosum
○ Extensive parakeratosis
○ Auspitz sign: Multiple, minute, bleeding points when the scale is lifted from the plaque (due to close proximity of dermal vessels to parakeratotic scale)
○ Munro micro abscesses: Neutrophils form small aggregates within the parakeratotic stratum corneum

Note
○ **Koebner phenomenon:** Psoriatic lesions can be induced in susceptible individuals by local trauma

Q5. Write a short note on lichen planus.
Ans.
Lichen planus
○ Self-limited disorder, resolves spontaneously in 1 to 2 years after onset
○ **Complication:** Squamous cell carcinoma in chronic lesions

Morphology
○ Pruritic, purple, polygonal, planar, papules, and plaques (6 Ps), seen on skin and mucosa
○ **Wickham striae:** White lacelike pattern of lines on papules
○ **Sites:** Extremities, wrists and elbows, glans penis

Microscopy
○ Acanthosis, hypergranulosis, hyperkeratosis
○ **Interface dermatitis:** Dense, continuous band-like infiltrate of lymphocytes along the dermoepidermal junction
○ Dermoepidermal interface shows angulated zigzag contour (sawtoothing)
○ Destruction of basal keratinocytes, which show degeneration, necrosis and shows squamatization
○ **Colloid or civatte bodies:** Anucleate, necrotic basal cells

Q6. Write a note on tuberculoid leprosy.
Ans.
Tuberculoid leprosy
○ Neuronal involvement dominates tuberculoid leprosy
○ Nerves become enclosed within granulomatous inflammatory reactions and are destroyed
○ Patient presents with dry, scaly skin lesions that lack sensation

○ There is asymmetric involvement of large peripheral nerves
○ As the host immune response is strong, with resultant granulomatous inflammation, lepra bacilli are never found on microscopic examination, hence it is termed paucibacillary leprosy

Q7. Write a note on lepromatous leprosy.

Ans.

Lepromatous leprosy

○ Severe form
○ Includes symmetric skin thickening and nodules
○ Mycobacterium invades into Schwann cells and into endoneural and perineural macrophages, with resultant damage of the peripheral nervous system
○ Can involve skin, peripheral nerves, anterior chamber of the eye, upper airways, testes, hands, and feet
○ Lesions contain macrophage aggregates which are filled with masses ("globi") of acid-fast bacilli
○ On face, nodular lesions coalesce to yield a distinctive **leonine facies**

25

Bone, Joints and Soft Tissue Tumors

Q 1. Write a note on Paget's disease of bone.

Ans.

Paget disease

○ Also called **osteitis deformans**

○ Disorder of increased bone mass

○ New bone deposition is disordered

○ Mutations in SQSTM1 gene is seen in Paget disease

○ Average age at diagnosis is 70 years

3 phases

a. Osteolytic stage

b. Mixed osteoclastic—osteoblastic stage, followed by predominant osteoblastic phase

c. Osteosclerotic stage

Morphology

○ Microscopic hallmark is **mosaic pattern of lamellar bone**, seen in the sclerotic stage

Q2. Write a note on fracture healing.

Ans.

Steps involved in fracture healing

1. At the site of fracture, there occurs hematoma formation, due to rupture of blood vessels

2. Due to the release of PDGF, TGF-α, FGF from inflammatory cells, there is deposition of uncalcified tissue, called procallus or soft tissue callus

3. After 2 weeks, soft tissue callus changes into bony callus

4. First woven bone is produced in the bony callus, which in two to three weeks time is replaced by lamellar bone

Complications: Non-union, malunion at the fracture site or pseudoarthrosis

Q3. Write a note on pyogenic osteomyelitis.

Ans.

Pyogenic osteomyelitis

Organisms may reach the bone by
- Hematogenous spread
- Extension from a contiguous site
- Direct implantation

Etiology
- *Staphylococcus aureus* is the most common responsible agent
- *Escherichia coli*, Pseudomonas, and Klebsiella are isolated from individuals with genitourinary tract infections or from intravenous drug abusers
- *Haemophilus influenzae* and group B streptococci are most common in neonates
- Sickle cell disease patients are predisposed to Salmonella infection

Morphology
- In acute phase, bacteria proliferate and induce a neutrophilic inflammatory reaction
- Necrosis of bone cells and marrow occurs within the first 48 hours
- Dead bone is called **sequestrum**
- A draining sinus can develop between the infected bone and the skin
- New bone deposition is seen as the time progresses, which is called **involucrum**

Q4. Write a note on cartilage-forming bone tumors.

Ans.

Cartilage-forming tumors

Behavior	Tumor type	Location
Benign	Osteochondroma	Metaphysis of long bones
	Chondroma	Small bones of hands and feet
	Chondroblastoma	Epiphysis of long bones
	Chondromyxoid fibroma	Tibia, pelvis
Malignant	Chondrosarcoma	Pelvis, shoulder

Q5. Write a note on osteochondroma in relation to its gross and microscopy.

Ans.

Osteochondroma (exostosis)
- Most common benign bone tumor
- Mostly **solitary**
- Can be a part of multiple **hereditary exostosis syndrome**
- **Site:** Arises from the metaphysis near the knee joint
- **Age group:** 10–30 years

Morphology

Gross

o Osteochondromas are sessile or pedunculated lesions, range in size from 1 to 20 cm

Microscopy

o Cartilage cap is composed of benign hyaline cartilage and has the appearance of disorganized growth plate
o Osteochondromas usually stop growing at the time of closure of growth plate

Q6. Discuss osteogenic sarcoma in relation to its etiology, radiological, clinical and morphological features.

Ans.

Etiopathogenesis of osteogenic sarcoma

o Malignant tumor in which the cancerous cells produce osteoid matrix or mineralized bone
o **Bimodal age distribution:** 75% patients are younger than 20 years of age, second peak occurs in older adults
o **Predisposing factors:** Paget disease, bone infarcts, and prior radiation
o Following mutations are noted in osteosarcoma: **RB** gene mutation, **TP53** gene mutation, **INK4a** inactivation

Clinical features

o **Site:** Metaphyseal region of long bones, most commonly around knee joint
o **Clinical features:** Painful, progressively enlarging mass or pathological fracture

Radiographic features of osteosarcoma

o Shows large destructive, mixed lytic and blastic mass with infiltrative margins
o Tumor breaks through the cortex and lifts the periosteum
o **Codman triangle**—triangular shadow between the cortex and raised ends of periosteum seen radiographically

Morphology

o **Most common subtype:** Arises from the metaphysis and is primary, intramedullary, osteoblastic, and high grade

Gross

o Tan-white tumor in metaphysis and proximal diaphysis
o Tumor infiltrates the cortex, lifts the periosteum, and form soft tissue masses on both sides of the bone

Microscopy

o Tumor cells vary in size and shape and have large hyperchromatic nuclei
o Bizarre tumor giant cells are common
o Formation of fine, lacelike pattern of neoplastic bone produced by the tumor cells is diagnostic
o Abnormal mitotic figures are also seen

Q7. Write a note on Ewing's sarcoma.

Ans.

Ewing sarcoma

○ Second most common sarcomas after osteosarcomas in children

Age group

○ Younger than 20 years, males are more commonly affected
○ **Site:** Diaphysis of long bones especially femur and flat bones of pelvis
○ **Clinical features:** Painful enlarging mass, fever, elevated erythrocyte sedimentation rate (ESR), anemia, and leukocytosis
○ **X-ray:** It shows a **destructive lytic tumor** with a characteristic periosteal reaction in which the layers of the reactive bone is deposited in onion-skin fashion
○ **Pathogenesis: t(11;22)** Translocation resulting in the fusion of the EWS gene on chromosome 22 to the FLI1 gene

Morphology

○ Composed of sheets of uniform small, round cells
○ Tumor cells have scant clear cytoplasm (clear as it is rich in **glycogen**)
○ Geographic necrosis may be prominent

Q8. Write a note on osteoclastoma (giant cell tumor).

Ans.

Giant cell tumor

○ Due to presence of multinucleated osteoclast-type giant cells, they are also called **osteoclastoma**
○ More common in females, age group: 20–40 years

Pathogenesis

○ Neoplastic cells of giant cell tumor are primitive osteoblast precursors
○ Tumor is comprised mainly of non-neoplastic osteoclasts
○ Neoplastic cells express high levels of RANKL, resulting in osteoclastic proliferation and hence resulting in destructive resorption of bone matrix

Site

○ Arises in the **epiphysis**, most commonly around knee joint (distal femur and proximal tibia)
○ Solitary, can be multicentric (in distal extremities)

X-ray

○ Lytic, expansile lesion in the epiphysis

Microscopy

○ Tumor comprises sheets of uniform oval mononuclear cells (neoplastic) and numerous osteoclast-type giant cells
○ Nuclei of the mononuclear cells and the osteoclasts are ovoid in shape with prominent nucleoli

Q9. Enumerate the differential diagnosis of giant cell tumor of bone.

Ans.

Differential diagnosis of giant cell tumor of bone

○ Chondroblastoma, metaphyseal fibrous defect, non-ossifying fibroma, chondromyxoid fibroma, Langerhans cell histiocytosis, solitary bone cyst, osteitis fibrosa cystica, aneurysmal bone cyst, giant cell reparative granuloma, osteoid osteoma, osteoblastoma

Q10. What is pannus?

Ans.

Pannus

○ In rheumatoid arthritis, destroyed joints are replaced by a mass (pannus) comprising of edematous synovial tissue, inflammatory cells, granulation tissue, and fibroblasts that grow over the articular cartilage

○ Pannus bridges the opposing bones, to form fibrous ankylosis, which over time ossifies and results in fusion of bones called bony ankylosis

Q11. Write a note on gout.

Ans.

Gout

○ Transient attacks of acute arthritis initiated by the deposition of monosodium urate crystals within and around joints

○ **Primary gout:** Unknown cause

○ **Secondary gout:** Uric acid is increased because of underlying disease (and disease predominates clinical picture)

Pathogenesis

○ **Hyperuricemia (plasma urate level above 6.8 mg/dl)** is necessary, but not sufficient, for development of gout

○ Hyperuricemia results from either overproduction or the reduced excretion of uric acid

Morphology

a. Acute arthritis

○ Dense neutrophilic infiltrate in the synovium

○ Monosodium urate crystals are found in the cytoplasm of neutrophils, which appear as long, slender, needle-shaped, and negatively birefringent

b. Chronic tophaceous arthritis

○ Repetitive precipitation of urate crystals during acute attacks

○ Synovium becomes hyperplastic, fibrotic, thickened and forms pannus

c. Tophi at various sites

○ Tophi are pathognomonic hallmark of gout

○ Aggregates of urate crystals surrounded by reactive fibroblasts, inflammatory cells, and giant cells

○ **Sites:** Articular cartilage, ligaments, tendons, bursae, earlobes, fingertips, skin

d. Gouty nephropathy
- ○ Urate crystals deposition in renal medullary interstitium or tubules
- ○ Uric acid nephrolithiasis and pyelonephritis

Q12. Write a note on liposarcoma.
Ans.

Liposarcoma
- ○ **Age group:** 50–60 years
- ○ **Sites:** Proximal extremities and in the retroperitoneum

Three morphologic subtypes
a. Well-differentiated liposarcoma
- ○ Shows mature adipocytes and scattered spindle cells with hyperchromatic nuclei
b. Myxoid liposarcoma
- ○ Proliferating lipoblasts in different stages of differentiation, prominent anastomosing capillary network and mucoid matrix
c. Pleomorphic liposarcoma
- ○ Sheets of anaplastic cells, bizarre nuclei and immature adipocytes (lipoblasts)
- ○ Shows S-100, actin and desmin positivity

Q13. Write a note on rhabdomyosarcoma.
Ans.

Rhabdomyosarcoma
- ○ Malignant mesenchymal tumor with skeletal muscle differentiation
- ○ **Subtypes:** Embryonal, alveolar and pleomorphic
- ○ **Alveolar and embryonal rhabdomyosarcoma:** Most common soft tissue sarcoma of childhood and adolescence

a. Embryonal rhabdomyosarcoma
- ○ Common in head and neck region
- ○ **Gross:** Soft gray infiltrative mass
- ○ **Microscopy:** Sheets of primitive round and spindle cells in a myxoid stroma. Rhabdomyoblasts with visible cross-striations may be present

b. Alveolar rhabdomyosarcoma
- ○ 10–25 years of age group
- ○ Most common in the extremities
- ○ Tumor cells are small, round, or oval and are firmly attached to fibrous strands (resembling pulmonary alveoli)
- ○ Tumor cells can detach themselves, resulting in alveolar or pseudoglandular appearance

c. Pleomorphic rhabdomyosarcoma
- ○ Seen predominantly in adults
- ○ Common in extremities especially thigh

○ Characterized by numerous large, multinucleated, bizarre eosinophilic tumor cells

○ Confirmed by myogenin positivity

Q14. Write a note on schwannoma.

Ans.

Schwannomas

○ Benign tumors that exhibit Schwann cell differentiation and often arise from peripheral nerves

○ Most common site—**cerebellopontine angle**

○ Associated with inactivating mutations in **NF2 gene** on **chromosome 22**

Morphology

○ Well-circumscribed, encapsulated masses that abut the associated nerve without invading it

Gross

○ Tumors form firm, gray masses

Microscopy

○ Antoni A areas (appear as densely eosinophilic)

○ Antoni B areas (appear as loose pale)

○ Verocay bodies (anuclear zones in between Antoni A areas)

Q15. Write a note on neurofibroma.

Ans.

Neurofibromas

○ Benign nerve sheath tumor

○ Composed of neoplastic Schwann cells admixed with perineural like cells, fibroblasts, mast cells, and spindle cells

Morphology

a. **Localized cutaneous neurofibroma**

○ Un-encapsulated nodular lesions, arise in the dermis and subcutaneous fat

b. **Diffuse neurofibroma**

○ Tumor cells diffusely infiltrate the dermis and subcutaneous connective tissue, entrapping the fat and appendage structures

c. **Plexiform neurofibroma**

○ Tumors grow within and expand the nerve fascicles

○ Bland spindle cells are admixed with wavy collagen bundles resembling carrot shavings

26

Central Nervous System

Q1. Write a note on Prion diseases.

Ans.

○ **Prions:** Abnormal forms of a cellular protein that cause rapidly progressive neurodegenerative disorders

Examples (in humans)

○ Creutzfeldt-Jakob disease
○ Gerstmann-Sträussler-Scheinker syndrome
○ Fatal familial insomnia
○ Kuru

Pathogenesis and Molecular Genetics

○ Degenerative disorders, caused by "spreading" of misfolded proteins
○ Disease occurs when PrP undergoes a conformational change from its normal α-helix-containing isoform (PrPc) to an abnormal β-pleated sheet isoform, usually termed PrPsc
○ Accumulation of PrPsc in neural tissue results in disease

How this accumulation is brought about?

○ α-helical PrPc may spontaneously shift to α-sheet PrPsc conformation, due to germ line PrP mutations
○ **Propagation:** PrPsc converts other molecules of PrPc into PrPsc, resulting in formation of PrPsc aggregates

Q2. Write a note on Creutzfeldt-Jakob disease.

Ans.

Creutzfeldt-Jakob disease (CJD)

○ Most common Prion disease
○ Familial forms are caused by mutations in PRNP
○ Age group: Seventh decade, with average survival of 7 months

Variant Creutzfeldt-Jakob disease
○ Most common in young adults
○ Due to consumption of bovine spongiform encephalopathy agent in contaminated foods or blood transfusion

Morphology
○ Pathognomonic finding: Spongiform transformation of the cerebral cortex

Microscopy
○ Small, microscopic empty vacuoles within the neuropil and in neurons
○ **Advanced cases:** Severe neuronal loss, reactive gliosis, expansion of vacuolated areas into cyst like spaces ("status spongiosus")

Q3. Write a note on Parkinson disease.
Ans.

Parkinson disease (PD)
○ Neurodegenerative disease characterized by prominent hypokinetic movement disorder

Etiology
○ Loss of dopaminergic neurons in the substantia nigra

Clinical features
○ Diminished facial expression (masked facies), stooped posture, slowing of voluntary movement, festinating gait (progressively shortened, accelerated steps), rigidity, and "pill-rolling" tremor
○ Triad of parkinsonism—tremor, rigidity, and bradykinesia

Molecular genetics and pathogenesis
a. α-synuclein aggregation results in autosomal dominant PD
   ○ α-synuclein aggregates are toxic to neurons
   ○ These aggregates have been termed Lewy bodies and Lewy neurites

Morphology
○ Characteristic finding is pallor of substantia nigra, due to loss of pigmented, catecholaminergic neurons
○ **Lewy bodies:** Single or multiple cytoplasmic, eosinophilic, round to elongated inclusions that often have a dense core surrounded by a pale halo
○ Lewy bodies are composed of **α-synuclein**

Q4. What are Negri bodies?
Ans.

Negri bodies
○ Pathognomonic microscopic finding in rabies
○ These are cytoplasmic, round to oval, eosinophilic inclusions
○ Found in pyramidal neurons of the hippocampus and Purkinje cells of the cerebellum

Q5. Write a note on cerebrospinal fluid (CSF) findings in pyogenic meningitis.

Ans.

CSF examination in pyogenic meningitis
- Appearance: turbid or purulent
- Leucocytes: Increased (>1000/microlitre), mainly neutrophils
- Proteins (mg/dl): Increased (50–1500)
- Glucose (mg/dl): Decreased (<40)

Q6. Write a note on cerebrospinal fluid (CSF) findings in tuberculous meningitis.

Ans.

CSF examination in tuberculous meningitis
- Appearance: Clear or cloudy
- Leucocytes: Increased (100–600/microliter), mainly lymphocytes
- Proteins (mg/dl): Increased (45–300)
- Glucose (mg/dl): Decreased (10–45)

Q7. Write a note on pilocytic astrocytoma.

Ans.

Pilocytic astrocytomas
- Seen in children and young adults
- **Site:** Cerebellum (most commonly) followed by optic chiasm and brainstem

Pathogenesis
- Associated with neurofibromin gene mutation, in NF-1 patients
- BRAF mutations

Morphology
- Tumors are often cystic
- Composed of bipolar cells with long, thin "hair like" processes, and shows GFAP-positivity
- Rosenthal fibers and eosinophilic granular bodies are seen

Q8. Write a note on glioblastoma multiforme.

Ans.

Glioblastoma (glioblastoma multiforme)

Sites
- Cerebral hemispheres in adults
- Cerebellum and brainstem in children

Salient features
- Cytoplasmic and nuclear pleomorphism, increased mitosis
- Vascular/endothelial cell proliferation producing glomeruloid like vessels (glomeruloid body), due to **VEGF** production by the **malignant astrocytes**
- **Geographic pattern of necrosis:** Tumor cells collect along the edges of the necrotic regions (**pseudo-palisading pattern**)

Q9. Write a note on medulloblastoma.

Ans.

Medulloblastoma (WHO grade IV)

- Most commonly affects children
- Most common site: Cerebellum

Molecular genetics

- Loss of chromosome 17p material
- MYC amplification is associated with aggressive clinical course

Morphology

Gross

- Well-circumscribed, gray, friable mass in the cerebellum

Microscopy

- Sheets of small cells with scant cytoplasm, ill-defined cell borders and hyperchromatic nuclei, which are angular or ovoid shape
- Mitosis are abundant
- Tumor cells can form Homer Wright rosettes and express GFAP positivity

Q10. Write a note on the morphology of meningiomas.

Ans.

Meningiomas

- Benign dural based tumors of adults, that arise from the meningothelial cells of arachnoid

Morphology

Gross

- Encapsulated, dural-based tumor
- Can spread in a sheet-like fashion along the dural surface

Microscopy: Following patterns are recognized

a. WHO Grade I/IV

- **Syncytial:** Whorled clusters of cells, with indistinct cell membranes, pseudo-inclusions, cellular whorls, psammoma bodies
- **Fibroblastic:** Spindle-shaped cells and a fascicular or storiform architecture
- **Transitional:** Features of syncytial and fibroblastic types
- **Psammomatous:** Composed of psammoma bodies, formed from the calcification of syncytial nests of meningothelial cells
- **Secretory:** PAS-positive intra-cytoplasmic droplets
- **Microcystic:** With a loose, spongy appearance

b. **Atypical meningiomas (WHO grade II/IV)**
   ○ Aggressive tumors
   ○ High rate of recurrence
   ○ **Examples:** Clear cell and chordoid meningioma

c. **Anaplastic (malignant) meningioma (WHO grade III/IV)**
   ○ Highly aggressive tumors
   ○ High mitotic rates (>20 mitoses per 10 high power fields)
   ○ **Examples:** Papillary and rhabdoid meningioma

Eye

Q1. Write a note on retinoblastoma.

Ans.

Retinoblastoma

- Most common primary intraocular malignancy of children
- Inherited cases: Occurs in individuals who inherit a germline mutation of one RB allele
- Sporadic cases: In individuals with no germline mutations and loss of Rb genes occurs following Knudson's two hit hypothesis

Morphology

- Tumor cells appear as collections of small, round cells with hyperchromatic nuclei
- Viable tumor cells are found encircling the blood vessels
- Flexner-Wintersteiner rosettes can be seen
- Foci of dystrophic calcification is a characteristic feature

Miscellaneous Questions

Q1. Write a note on fine needle aspiration cytology.

Ans.

Fine needle aspiration cytology
- It is a diagnostic procedure used to investigate lumps or masses
- Performed by using a thin (22–25 gauge) needle
- Needle is inserted into a mass or nodule and the tissue cells are aspirated with or without application of suction
- Tissue which is aspirated are smeared on a slide
- These slides are now stained with May-Grünwald Giemsa and Pap stain and are evaluated under the microscope for making a diagnosis

Q2. Write a note on exfoliative cytology.

Ans.
- In exfoliative cytology, cells shed from the body surfaces are collected and examined

How are the cells collected?

a. Spontaneous exfoliation
- Done in the cases of peritoneal fluid, pleural fluid, pericardial fluid, urine, cysts, washings (peritoneal, bladder), where the cells spontaneously shed into these washings are examined

b. Mechanical exfoliation
- Cells are manually scraped/brushed off the surface
- Done in cervical Pap smear and brushings (bronchial, gastric, biliary, oral, etc)

Note
- A brushing sample should be taken before a biopsy as the later results in bleeding and will obscure the brushing cells morphology

Q3. Write a note on erythrocyte sedimentation rate (ESR).

Ans.

Erythrocyte sedimentation rate (ESR)
- Measures the rate of settling (sedimentation) of erythrocytes

Comprises three stages
- **Stage 1:** Formation of rouleaux in which RBCs stack together like a pack of coins (10 minutes)
- **Stage 2:** Stage of sedimentation: In which rouleaux settles down (40 minutes)
- **Stage 3:** Packing of the rouleaux (10 minutes)

Factors affecting ESR
a. Factors increasing ESR
- Old age, pregnancy, anemia, elevated fibrinogen, macrocytosis, high temperature

b. Factors decreasing ESR
- Microcytosis, low fibrinogen, polycythemia, leucocytosis

Methods for estimation
- Westergren method
- Wintrobe method
- Zeta sedimentation ratio
- Micro-ESR method

Q4. Write a note on proteinuria.

Ans.
- Normal kidney can excrete up to 150 mg/24 hours of protein in urine
- **Proteinuria:** Protein excretion in urine greater than 150 mg/24 hours in adults

Causes of proteinuria
- **Glomerular proteinuria:** Can be selective (albumin and transferrin) and non-selective (large molecular weight proteins)
- **Tubular proteinuria:** Seen in acute pyelonephritis, chronic pyelonephritis, tuberculosis, heavy metal poisoning, interstitial nephritis, transplant rejection
- **Overflow proteinuria:** Seen in multiple myeloma (Bence Jones proteins), intravascular hemolysis (hemoglobin)
- **Hemodynamic proteinuria:** Transient and seen in patients with high fever, hypertension, heavy exercise, heart failure, seizures

Q5. Write a note on significance of the casts in urine.

Ans.
Renal casts
- Cylindrical, cigar-shaped structures, formed in the distal renal tubules and collecting ducts
- Casts are specifically of renal origin
- Composed of a precipitate of a protein secreted by the tubules (Tamm-Horsfall protein)

Two main types

a. Non-cellular: Hyaline, granular, waxy, fatty

b. Cellular: Red blood cell, white blood cell, renal tubular epithelial cell

Important points

○ Waxy casts: Seen in end stage renal failure

○ Fatty casts: Seen in nephrotic syndrome

○ Broad casts: Seen in chronic renal failure and renal tubular obstruction, associated with poor prognosis

○ Red cell casts: Indicate acute glomerulonephritis

○ White cell casts: Indicates pyelonephritis

○ Renal tubular epithelial cell casts: Seen in acute tubular necrosis, heavy metal poisoning, allograft rejection

Q6. Mention significance of ketone bodies in urine.

Ans.

○ Excretion of ketone bodies, i.e. acetoacetic acid, beta hydroxyl butyric acid and acetone in urine is termed ketonuria

○ Ketones are the breakdown products of fatty acids

○ Normally, ketone bodies are not detectable in urine, however, in individuals in whom fat is used as a source of energy, this fat breakdown is responsible for excessive production of ketone bodies

Conditions associated

a. Decreased utilization of carbohydrates as seen in diabetes mellitus with ketoacidosis

b. Decreased availability of carbohydrates: Seen in starvation, persistent vomiting

c. Glycogen storage disorders: von Gierke's disease

d. Increased metabolic needs: Fever, thyrotoxicosis, pregnancy

Q7. Mention four indications of bone marrow aspiration.

Ans.

Indications for bone marrow aspiration

○ Unexplained cytopenias

○ Suspected acute leukemia for classification and categorization

○ Suspected chronic myeloproliferative disorders

○ Suspected myelodyspalstic syndromes

○ Metastatic tumors to the marrow

○ Investigation of pyrexia of unknown origin

○ Suspected storage disorder like Gaucher's disease or Neimann-Pick disease

○ Suspected infections like kala-azar, miliary tuberculosis, or histoplasmosis

Indications for bone marrow biopsy
○ Dry tap as seen in myelofibrosis or leukemia
○ Suspected aplastic anemia
○ Suspected myelofibrosis
○ Suspected hairy cell leukemia
○ Staging of lymphoma

Q8. Write a note on Bombay blood group.

Ans.

Bombay blood group
○ H-gene produces a transferase enzyme
○ Transferase changes precursor substance into H substance on the RBC surface
○ H-substance is converted into A and B antigens by A and B genes (present on chromosome 9) on RBC surface
○ Some individuals do not inherit H gene (genotype hh) and thus cannot synthesize H substance
○ Such individuals may inherit A or B gene but cannot express as they are not converted to A and B antigens
○ These individuals are said to have Bombay phenotype or Bombay blood group
○ They lack H, A and B antigens and their red cells type as group O
○ It is an extremely rare blood group and is not compatible with any of the blood groups on crossmatching

Q9. Write a note on blood components prepared in blood bank.

Ans.

Blood components
○ Red cells: Packed red cells, leucocyte—poor red cells, washed red cells, frozen red cells, irradiated red cells
○ Platelets: Platelet concentrate, apheresis platelets
○ Granulocyte concentrate

Plasma components
○ Fresh frozen plasma
○ Cryoprecipitate

Q10. Discuss the principle of crossmatching.

Ans.

Crossmatching
○ **Aim:** To prevent the transfusion of incompatible red cell units
○ **Two types:** Major crossmatch and minor crossmatch
○ **Major crossmatch:** Testing the recipient serum against donor red cells
○ **Minor crossmatch:** Testing the donor serum against recipient red cells

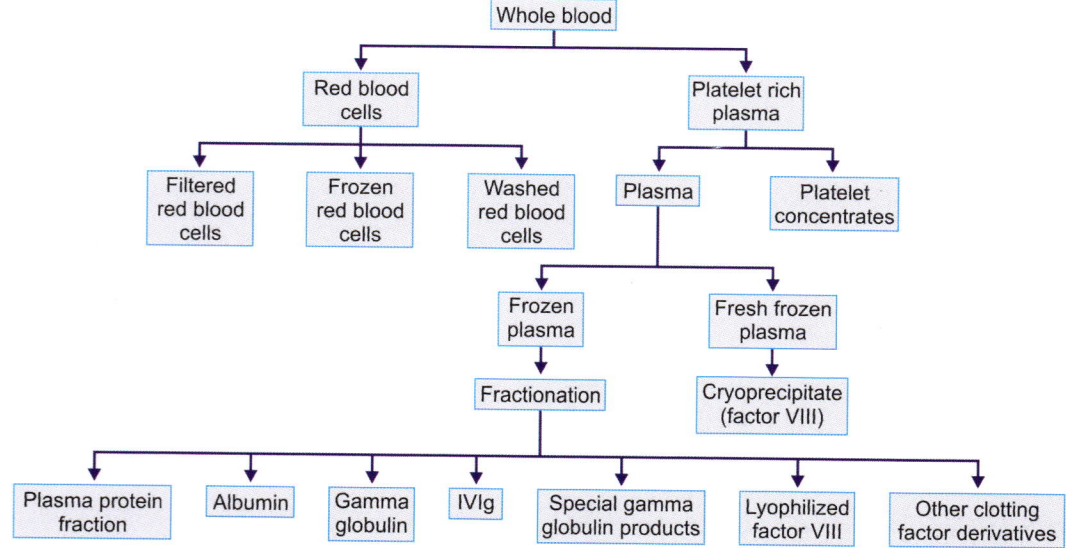

Fig. 28.1: Blood components separation

Note

○ **Minor crossmatch** is not important and therefore, only the red blood cells from the donor unit are tested against the recipient serum

○ For transfusion of platelets or fresh frozen plasma, crossmatching is not required

Q11. Write a note on reticulocyte count in relation to its procedure and interpretation.

Ans.

Reticulocytes

○ Are young RBCs containing remnants of RNA and ribosomes

○ Recognized by supravital stains which detect RNA in these cells

○ RNA appears as blue precipitating granules within RBCs

○ Supravital staining refers to staining of these cells in a living state

Principle

○ A few drops of blood are incubated with methylene blue solution which stains granules of RNA in red cells

Reagent

New methylene blue solution is prepared as follows:

○ New methylene blue: 1gm

○ Sodium citrate: 0.6 gm

○ Sodium chloride: 0.7 gm

○ Distilled water: 100 ml

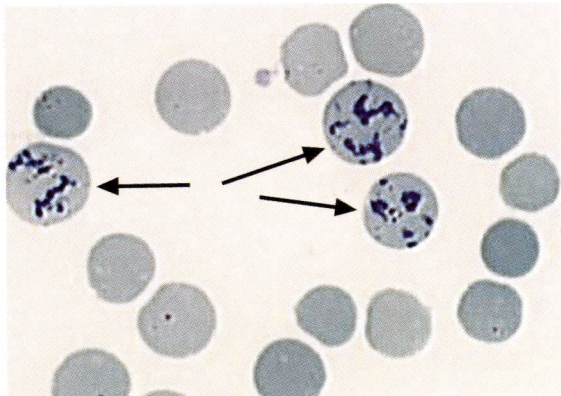

Fig. 28.2: Reticulocytes (demonstrated by arrow)

Reagent should be kept stored in a refrigerator at 2–6 degree celsius and filtered before use

Other dyes used include: Brilliant cresyl blue and azure B

Sample
○ EDTA blood sample

Method
1. In a test tube, take 2–3 drops of filtered new methylene blue solution
2. Add equal amount of blood and mix well
3. Keep the mixture at room temperature for 15 minutes
4. Prepare a smear from the small drop of mixture prepared above
5. Slide should be viewed under oil immersion lens in a microscope
6. Reticulocytes show deep blue precipitates in the red blood cells

Result
○ Number of reticulocyte is expressed as a percentage of red cells

Reference range
○ Reticulocyte percentage: 0.5 – 2.5%

Index